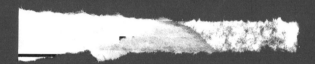

DONKEYS
Miniature, Standard, and Mammoth
A Veterinary Guide for Owners and Breeders

STEPHEN R. PURDY, DVM

Foreword by Paul and Betsy Hutchins, Founders,
The American Donkey and Mule Society

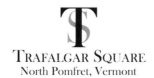

TRAFALGAR SQUARE
North Pomfret, Vermont

Dedication

For my parents, Clyde Nelson Purdy and Maisie Carpenter Purdy, who were dedicated to each other, their children, and their family.

First published in 2010 by
Trafalgar Square Books
North Pomfret, Vermont 05053

Printed in Hong Kong, China

Library of Congress Cataloging-in-Publication Data

Purdy, Stephen R.
  Donkeys : miniature, standard, and mammoth : a veterinary guide for owners and breeders / Stephen R. Purdy.
    p. cm.
  Includes bibliographical references and index.
  ISBN 978-1-57076-418-9
  1. Donkeys. I. Title.
  SF361.P87 2009
  636.1'82--dc22
                          2009041240

Photo Credits:
All photos and illustrations courtesy of Dr. Stephen R. Purdy except: 1.1, 1.2, 1.4 (Nora Matthews); 1.4 A & B (Lynn Gattari); 4.7, 6.1, 6.2, 6.3, 7.1 (Linda Cunningham); 7.3, 7.5 (Michael Walker)

Book design by Erika Gavin
Cover design by R. M. Didier
Typeface: Scala Sans

10 9 8 7 6 5 4 3 2 1

Contents

Foreword

This is truly an outstanding book for the donkey owner. Whether you have one donkey or a large breeding farm, *Donkeys: Miniature, Standard, and Mammoth* belongs in your library. What a help it would have been to have had this book when we started the American Donkey and Mule Society! The lack of such a reference was a need that every donkey owner and veterinarian can be grateful to have now had filled.

Dr. Steve Purdy obviously has studied and put to practical use his knowledge of the care, breeding, feeding, and treatment of donkeys. The information he provides is well founded in science and detailed in nature without being too scientific for the average donkey owner to understand. His ability to make the information clear and easy to use is one of the best features of this book.

We highly recommend that everyone who deals with donkeys in any capacity—from pet or rescue, to breeding and veterinary work—buy this book and read it carefully.

Paul and Betsy Hutchins
Founders, The American Donkey and Mule Society
Authors, *The Definitive Donkey*

Acknowledgments

There are many people who have influenced me and helped me become the person and veterinarian I am today. I thank my father and mother, Clyde Nelson Purdy and Maisie Carpenter Purdy, not only for their DNA but also for their positive support throughout my life. They taught me that anything is possible and, by their example, the value of hard work and doing the right thing. Service to others and to a "higher cause" was the norm in our home growing up and so is a large part of my life today.

My paternal grandparents, Clyde Ransley Purdy and Edna Sleator Purdy, inspired me in the same way. Their love and support was never in question. My maternal grandmother Anna Kaiser Carpenter lived to be 100 years old. She was an inspiration to our whole family.

I also thank my brother Thomas Edward Purdy, and sister JoAnn Purdy, for their friendship and love. My children, Cooper Nelson Southworth-Purdy and Greer Veronica Southworth-Purdy, have been the delight of my life. Parenting is the most difficult task I have undertaken, and as it is said, "It never ends." The rewards are enormous.

I also wish to acknowledge my teachers—reaching back to high school—who demonstrated the importance of excellence. Among many I note in particular Jean Walker, Robert Bragg, and Matt Farnum. Scott Sanford was my high school coach and a very strong positive influence in my life. In veterinary school I owed a great deal to my teachers. Many inspired me and continue to do so today, including Francis Fox, Susan Fubini, Normand Ducharme, and William Hornbuckle. My greatest influence as a practicing veterinarian continues to be Edwin Mackey. I met Dr. Mackey and his wonderful family before I applied to veterinary school. They treated me as they did everyone—as a member of the family. Jean and Ed Mackey were, to me, models of service to animals and animal owners. Dr. Mackey was a true renaissance man and the most intelligent veterinarian I have ever met. When I found myself in some difficult situation during my full-time practice years, I often thought, "What would Doc Mackey do?" "His best," was always the answer.

I thank my students Carolyn Emery, PJ Stanley, and Weston Brown, and the excellent artist and friend Linda Cunningham for their contributions. I also thank veterinarians Nora Matthews, Michael Walker, and Tex Taylor for their invaluable help. In conclusion thank you to everyone at Trafalgar Square Books for their advice, and corrections, additions, and subtractions to this book.

The History of the Donkey

Introduction

Donkey is the common name for the members of the species *Equinis asinus*, more correctly called the ass. The name donkey comes from an old English word "dunkey" meaning an animal that is grayish brown in color.[1] The ancestors of the modern donkey are the Nubian and Somalian subspecies of African Wild Ass,[2,3] which was domesticated around 4,000 BC. The donkey became an important pack animal for people living in the Egyptian and Nubian regions as they can easily carry 20–30% of their own body weight and can also be used as a farming and dairy animal. By 1,800 BC, the ass had reached the Middle East, where the trading city of Damascus was referred to as the "City of Asses." Syria produced at least three breeds of donkeys, including a saddle breed with a graceful, easy gait.[4]

For the Greeks, the donkey was associated with the Syrian god of wine, Dionysus. The Romans also valued the ass and originally introduced it to the British Isles. Equines had become extinct in the Western Hemisphere at the end of the last Ice Age. However, horses and donkeys were reintroduced to the Americas by the Spanish Conquistadors. In 1495, the ass first appeared in the New World when Christopher Columbus introduced four jacks (males) and two jennies (females). This bloodline produced many of the mules that the Conquistadors used while they explored the Americas. Shortly after America became independent, George Washington imported the first Mammoth Jack stock into the country. Because the existing jack donkeys in the New World lacked the size and strength needed to produce quality work mules, he imported donkeys from Spain and France, some standing over 1.63 meters (16 hands) tall. One of the donkeys, "Knight of Malta," that Washington received stood 1.43 meters (14 hands) and was regarded as a great disappointment. Viewing this donkey as unfit for producing mules, Washington instead used Knight of Malta for cross-breeding to develop desirable qualities. This led to

1.1 Tethered in Morocco.

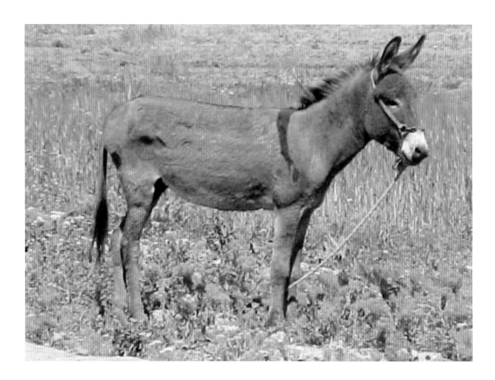

the American line of Mammoth Jacks (a breed name that includes both males and females) with size and substance preferred for siring mules.[5]

Despite these early appearances in America, the donkey did not find widespread distribution until it was found to be useful as a pack animal by miners, particularly gold prospectors of the mid-1800s. Miners preferred this animal for its ability to carry tools, supplies, and ore. The donkey's sociable disposition and adaptation to human companionship allowed miners to lead them without ropes as they simply followed behind their owner. As mining became less an occupation for the individual prospector and more of an industrialized, underground operation, the miners' donkeys lost their jobs and many were turned loose into the American deserts. Descendants of these donkeys, now feral, roam the Southwest today.[6]

By the early twentieth century, donkeys began to be used less as working animals and instead were kept as pets in the United States and other affluent nations while remaining an important work animal in many poorer parts of the world. The donkey as a pet is best portrayed by the appearance of the miniature donkey in 1929 when they were imported to the United States by Robert Green, a lifetime advocate of the breed. Mr. Green is best quoted when he said, "Miniature donkeys possess the affectionate nature of a Newfoundland, the resignation of a cow, the durability of a mule, the courage of a tiger, and the intellectual capability only slightly inferior to man's."[7]

Global Importance

In Ethiopia, a donkey costs at least half the annual family income. It is considered the most important possession a family can own. If not for the donkey, most families would not be able to support themselves; such is the importance of the donkey worldwide. There are approximately 90 million donkeys at work in third-world nations, including Tunisia, Ethiopia, Egypt, Turkey, Peru, Mexico, Costa Rica, and Morocco. Their contribution to farming and the basic economy of such countries is enormous. The donkey is the workhorse that powers the subsistence-based agricultural industry that supports the populations of every inhabited continent in the world.

Nutrition and basic husbandry of donkeys are important as the welfare of the family depends on the health of the donkey(s) owned. It is interesting to note that the donkeys owned by a rural family are most often cared for by the women. If not for the donkey, the women become beasts of burden, whereupon they weaken under the work load and may sicken and die, with a devastating impact on the family unit. In Ethiopia, when a donkey dies, the women cling together and weep.

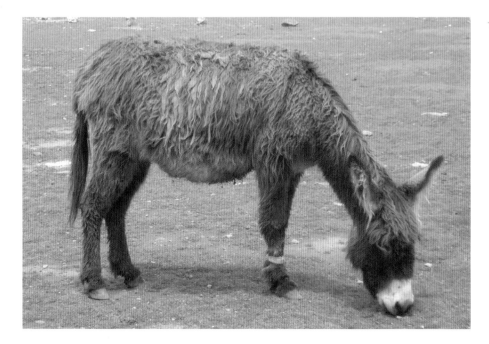

1.2 Hobbled in Peru.

Today, as the world becomes a smaller place, there is a call for better care for one of humanity's greatest allies in the struggle for daily survival. Healthy donkeys mean healthier children in the families that use them to cultivate their land. These people are eager to learn better techniques for keeping their donkeys healthy longer and living productive lives because family survival depends upon these animals. It is only in the industrialized nations of the Western world where donkeys are kept as pets; everywhere else in the world they are an integral part of the economic structure.

Reproduction is an important part of donkey ownership. Donkeys are carefully bred to produce strong, long-lived work animals that are valued as contributing members of the family within which they live. Subjects such as artificial insemination, reproductive health of the jennet, and foaling information are important topics of field education for third-world nations.

Research, both lab-based and field, is needed to bring donkey breeding and management to an efficient level to meet the needs of third-world populations that are dependent on subsistence agriculture.

1.3 Pulling a cart in Morocco.

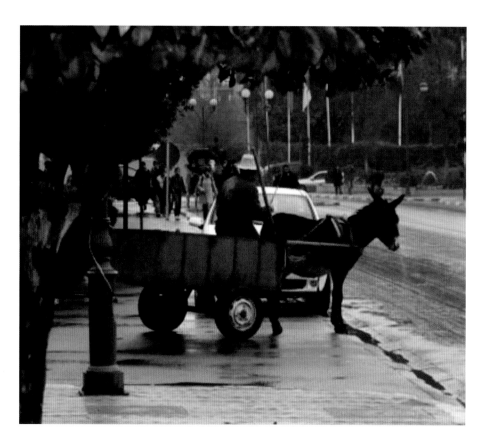

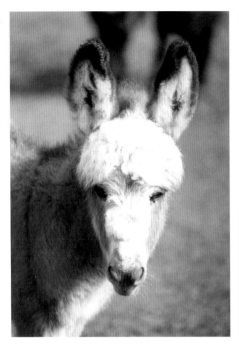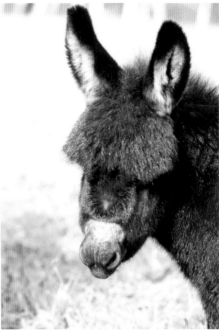

1.4 A & B Two Miniature Mediterranean Donkeys, from Dewey Meadows Farm, bred and born in Rome, New York.

Summary

- Donkey is the common name for the members of the species *Equinis asinus*, more correctly called the ass.

- The ancestors of the modern donkey are the Nubian and Somalian subspecies of African Wild Ass, which was domesticated around 4,000 BC.

- Despite early appearances in America, the donkey did not find widespread distribution until it was discovered to be useful as a pack animal by miners, particularly gold prospectors of the mid-1800s.

- There are approximately 90 million donkeys at work in third-world nations. Their contribution to farming and the basic economy of such countries is enormous.

- The donkey is the workhorse that powers the subsistence-based agricultural industry that supports the populations of every inhabited continent in the world.

- Donkeys are carefully bred to produce strong, long-lived work animals that are valued as contributing members of the family within which they live.

References

1. Agriculture and Food: Roping the Web: The official site of Agriculture, Food and Rural Development (AFRD) of Alberta Canada; www.agric.gov.ab.ca.

2. Clutton-Brook, J. *A Natural History of Domesticated Mammals.* Cambridge, UK, Cambridge University Press,1999.

3. Beja-Pereira, Albano et al. "African Origins of the Domestic Donkey." *Science.* 18 June 2004:Vol. 304. no. 5678, p. 1781.

4. Wikipedia, the free encyclopedia; http://en.wikipedia.org.

5. See note 4 above.

6. See note 4 above.

7. See note 4 above.

A Donkey Is Not a Horse

Nomenclature

- Donkey: worldwide common name for the ass family.
- Jack, jack Ass, or jackass: an intact male of the ass family.
- Jennet, jenny: the female of the ass family.
- Burro: a smaller member of the ass family, usually of Mexican or Spanish descent. Usually gray in color and commonly thought of as feral asses in the southwestern United States.
- Donkey gelding, or gelded jack: castrated male of the ass family.
- Mare: female horse.
- Stallion: intact (un-neutered) male horse.
- Jack stock: animals of mammoth size regardless of sex; similar to the term "cattle" for cows.
- Hybrid crosses:
  Hinny—the hybrid cross resulting from breeding a stallion to a jenny.
  Mule—the hybrid cross resulting from breeding a mare to a jack.
- Miniature donkey: member of the donkey family that stands at 36 inches or less at the withers at maturity.
- Standard donkey: between 36 and 54 inches (9–13.2 hands) at the withers at maturity.
- Mammoth donkey: greater than 54 inches (13.2 hands) at the withers at maturity.[1]

Genetic Makeup

Domestic horses have 64 chromosomes, the domestic ass has 62, and the mule and hinny each have 63. Both hybrid crosses are considered sterile even though there are documented cases of fertility in the female mule. There are no documented cases of fertility in either the female hinny or male of the cross created by breeding a stallion to a jenny. Spermatozoa are not produced in the testes of male mules because of incompatibility between paternal and maternal chromosomes; this blocks the halving of chromosomes (meiosis) during cell division of a developing, fertilized egg. The same chromosomal incompatibility causes partial arrest of meiosis in female mules and hinnies with subsequent and severe depletion of oocytes (eggs) at birth.

Female mules and hinnies can be used as embryo recipients. They do have estrus cycles, but these are often erratic. Male mules are not seasonal in behavior and therefore may be used as teasers to determine when mares or jennets are in estrus. It is possible to train mares to accept pasture breeding by a jack, but it is not always successful.

Anatomic Differences: Donkeys, Horses, and Mules

Ear length of donkeys is usually greater than in mules, which, in turn, have longer ears than horses. It should be noted that many donkey and mule withers cannot hold a saddle well because they are relatively rounded as com-

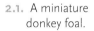

2.1. A miniature donkey foal.

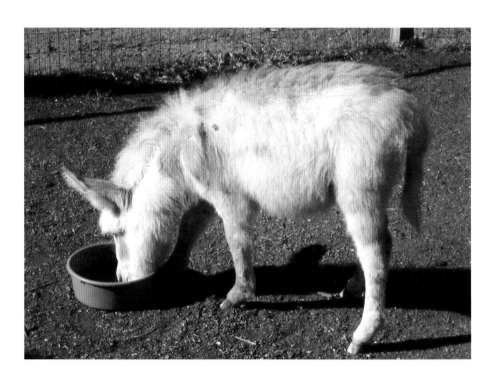

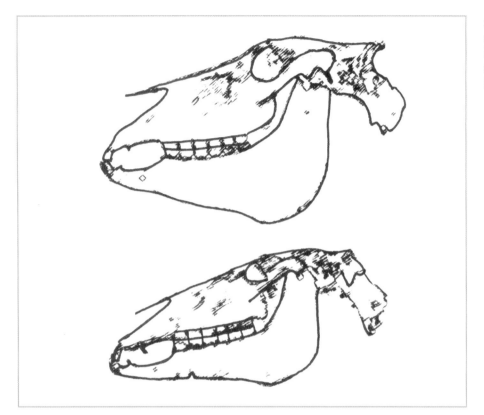

2.2 The comparison of skull size between a 450 kg (1,000 lb) donkey (top) and the same weight horse (bottom).

pared to the horse. The donkey's mane and tail hair is stiff and its tail has short hair, whereas mule tails may be more like horses. The donkey's croup (buttock) muscles are usually less developed than those of horses.

Obvious differences in the shape of the donkey and horse skulls are evident in fig. 2.3. The donkey pelvis tips down and back more than the horse. This is important as it relates to techniques used for reproductive exams and dystocias (difficult births). Donkey hooves are smaller than those for equal-sized horses, with the frog set more toward the heel than it is in the horse (figs. 2.3 A & B). The pastern angles for donkeys are more upright than those of a horse. Donkeys do not have chestnuts in the rear legs as horses do. In mules, rear chestnuts may be absent or smaller as compared to horses.

It can be difficult to draw blood from a donkey's jugular vein if using the same technique as with the horse. The donkey jugular vein is not palpable throughout the neck because the middle third is covered by a thick cutaneous coli muscle.[2] A sample is more readily obtained by a needle puncture in the upper or lower one-third of the jugular groove.

2.3 A & B A miniature donkey's front foot (A) and hind foot (B).

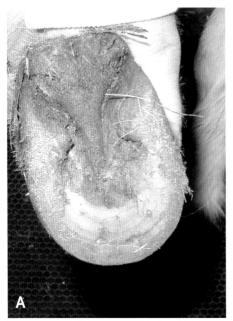 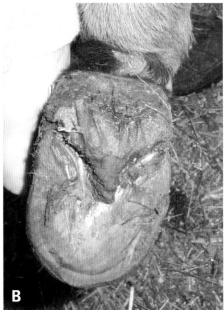

The donkey's respiratory system, and in particular the anatomy of the larynx, is slightly different from that of the horse. The nasal passages of donkeys and mules are smaller than those for equal-sized horses, necessitating the use of smaller nasogastric tubes when "tubing" animals to decompress the stomach or administer medication such as in colic (abdominal pain) situations. The nasolacrimal duct is the overflow pathway for tears. An opening at the inside corner of the eye runs through the skull to terminate at the end of the inside of the nose. In the donkey, the nasal opening is located inside the outside flare of the nostril, slightly toward the top, while in the horse this opening is found on the inside floor at the end of the nostril where the nasal skin and mucous membranes meet.

Medical Differences

Sedation and Anesthesia

Sedation with xylazine, butorphanol, or detomidine is appropriate for donkeys and the amount of drug used may also be diluted with sterile water or saline to increase the volume administered and thereby to allow for more accurate dosing. Various combinations of xylazine—0.6–1.0 mg/kg, IV (intravenously) or IM (intramuscularly)—with acepromazine (0.1 mg/kg, IV or IM) or butorphanol (0.02–0.04 mg/kg IV), or the use of detomidine (0.005–0.02 mg/kg, IV or IM) with butorphanol have been used with relatively good success, either for standing procedures (combined with local anesthesia) or before general anesthesia.[3] Miniature donkeys tend to require doses at the high end of these ranges.

One method for induction of general anesthesia prior to maintenance on gas, or for use alone for a short surgical procedure such as castration, is to sedate with xylazine (1.1 mg/kg, IV) and then induce general anesthesia with ketamine (2.2 mg/kg, IV). The addition of butorphanol (0.01–0.02 mg/kg, IV) or diazepam (0.03 mg/kg, IV) provides additional sedation and muscle relaxation. These drugs generally allow for 15 to 20 minutes of anesthesia in most donkeys. However, miniature donkeys are inadequately anesthetized even for a short procedure with these drug doses; they experience muscle rigidity and excitatory effects. I have achieved satisfactory results on miniature donkeys by increasing the dose rates for equal sized horses by 25% for xylazine, ketamine, and butorphanol.

Drug Metabolism

Research in the area of drug metabolism in donkeys is limited. We do know that differences exist among horses, donkeys, and mules, and possibly among different sizes of donkeys. It is difficult to make specific dosage and frequency recommendations for donkeys and for mules; most often horse doses are used for these animals. Since donkeys metabolize nonsteroidal anti-inflammatory drugs (NSAIDs) at different rates than horses, these medications need to be administered at different intervals than in the horse. Phenylbutazone [5] and flunixin meglumine [6] are more rapidly metabolized and may need to be given twice daily to standard donkeys and three times daily to miniature donkeys.[7]

The rapid metabolism of trimethoprim-sulfamethoxazole (TMS) given IV may make it inappropriate to use for antibacterial therapy in donkeys or mules. I suggest giving the dose of TMS orally twice daily.[8]

Behavioral Differences

Donkeys are very stoic when it comes to showing outward signs of pain. This

2.4 Poitou donkey yearlings.

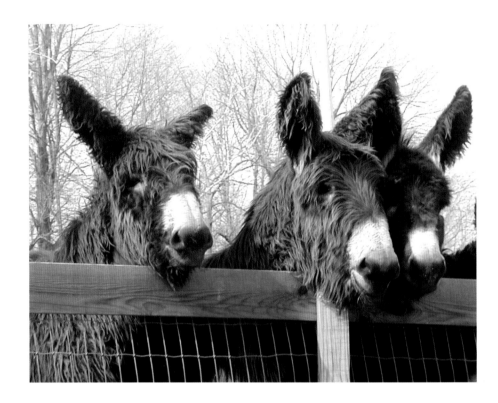

may be detrimental to early diagnosis and treatment of abnormalities. For example, a colic situation may go undetected until it is in more advanced stages so you should assume the presence of a severe problem when a donkey displays even mild signs of pain. An increased pulse rate is not always reliable in a donkey as a sign of a severe problem. Owners and veterinarians should look for subtle changes in behavior or attitude. This is best appreciated by knowing the normal behavior of individual animals. For example, you should assume that a donkey that will not eat is fairly sick, especially if the animal refuses grain. Standard colic treatment with decompression of the stomach, analgesics (pain relievers), and antacids should be administered early. (See the discussion of colic in chapter 6, p. 76.)

As another example, the stoicism of donkeys may allow laminitis to progress to a dangerous degree of circulatory damage in the foot without the animal showing severe signs of lameness. Donkeys are generally less responsive to hoof tester pressure across the sole than are horses. It is suggested that radiographs be taken early in the course of a laminitis case to look for rotation and/or sinking of the third phalanx (coffin bone or P3). (See the discussion of laminitis in chapter 7, p. 95.)

Tolerance of Medical Procedures

Medical procedures are best performed with other animals nearby to alleviate anxiety. This is not different from horses but is especially important in the donkey. For all their stoicism, donkeys are very sensitive to social or environmental changes. They need to see what is going on for a while before being asked to move to an unfamiliar location or being approached by unfamiliar equipment. What has been termed as "stubbornness" is actually a donkey's method of evaluating any novel situation: they do not like to rush into anything new. Their stop-and-back "gears" are well developed and they are also known to sit down when refusing to move into a new area such as an unfamiliar barn or onto a different surface, especially when moving from bright sunlight to a shaded area. A humane nose twitch works well in most donkeys for minor restraint. The general rule with donkeys is to "go slow and stay quiet."

Social Behavior

Donkeys are highly social animals and they form strong attachments to other animals of their own or other species with which they have been cohabitating. Jacks are often very aggressive toward newly introduced jennets when they first meet. The jack may need to wear a breeding muzzle for approximately half an hour on initial introduction to a new jennet, particularly when he is first turned out for pasture breeding. This aggressive behavior may also occur when he is returned to a herd after only a short separation. The muzzle may be removed after aggression calms down. Usually, the norm is for both jacks and jennets to initially display kicking, biting, and chasing behavior.

Vocalization is very common in donkeys. This is most often called "braying" although the uninitiated have described it as sounding like blood curdling screaming and torture. In general, braying is used as a greeting, or for demonstrating the emotions of being hungry or sexually interested. Breeding animals and jennets may call out to other jacks or jennets and donkeys greet their human caretakers at feeding time or in an attempt to beg for more food. Beware of letting your donkey become obese (see p. 22)!

Suggested Reading

- Hutchins, Betsy and Paul. *The Definitive Donkey: A Textbook on the Modern Ass.* Hee Haw Book Service, Lewisville, TX, 1999.
- Svendsen, E.D. *The Professional Handbook of the Donkey.* Whittet Books, Ltd, London,1997.

Because pecking order is important at feeding time, animals need sufficient space to eat, particularly in the winter in cold climates. Overweight animals may need to be housed in separate feeding groups to prevent obesity and to avoid starvation in timid or smaller animals.

Mothers correct foals early in life with mild kicking and biting. They may even "reward" a playful foal with a clamping bite on top of the head once they reach their limit of tolerance. The offending juvenile may then sulk but hopefully learns better behavior for the future. Foals "play fight" with mothers as early as on the day of birth. Mothers often move off from the herd to foal, and initially will keep newborns away from others. They may remain out in the rain or snow with a new foal rather than going inside. You may need to bring the foal in to encourage the pair to join the rest of the group. The jennet may be more at ease if penned adjacent to other animals in clear sight. Her antisocial behavior does not often last for long (see chapter 8 for more on reproduction).

Summary

- Donkey- and mule-specific terminology must be understood to speak intelligently to owners.

- Genetic makeup of donkeys, mules, and horses is different. Some interbreeding is possible. Most donkey/horse hybrids are sterile but females may cycle like horses.

- Several clinically important anatomical differences exist between donkeys and horses.

- Donkey behavior must be understood in order to handle them effectively and safely.

- Stoicism is manifested by disguising pain. Subtle differences in attitude and behavior may be the only indicators of severe problems.

- Social interaction is important to donkeys with regards to nutrition and reproduction.

- Drug metabolism is different among donkeys, horses, and mules. More research is needed to define correct dosage levels and intervals.

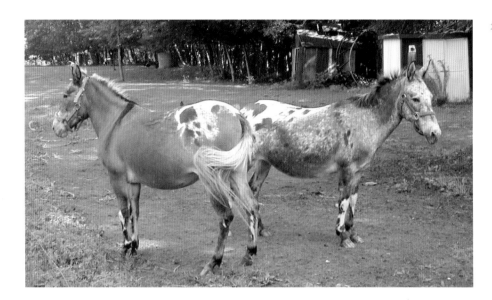

Appaloosa Hinnies.

References

1. Taylor, TS; Matthews, NS; Blanchard, TL. "Introduction to Donkeys in the US." *New England Journal of Large Animal Health*; 1(1): 21-28, 2001.

2. Burnham, SL. "Anatomical Differences of the Donkey and Mule." American Association of Equine Practitioners Proceedings 48:102-109, 2002.

3. Matthews, NS; Van Dijk, P. "Anesthesia and Analgesia for Donkeys." *Veterinary Care for Donkeys*, International Veterinary Information Service, Ithaca, NY (www.ivis.org), 2004.

4. See note 3 above.

5. Mealey, KL; Matthews, NS; Peck, KE, et al. "Comparative pharmacokinetics of phenylbutazone and its metabolite oxyphenbutazone in clinically normal horses and donkeys." *American Journal of Veterinary Research*. 1997; 58:53-55.

6. Coakley, M; Peck, KE; Taylor, TS; et al. "Pharmacokinetics of flunixin meglumine in donkeys, mules and horses." *American Journal of Veterinary Research*. 1999; 60:1441-1444.

7. Matthews, NS; Peck, KE; Taylor, TS; Mealey, KL. "Pharmacokinetics of Phenylbutazone and Its Metabolite Oxyphenbutazone in Miniature Donkeys." *American Journal of Veterinary Research*. 62(5): 673-675, 2001.

8. Peck, KE; Matthews, NS; Taylor, TS; Mealey, KL. "Pharmacokinetics of Sulfamethoxazole and Trimethoprim in Donkeys, Mules, and Horses." *American Journal of Veterinary Research*. 63(3): 349-353, 2002.

Nutrition

Introduction

The donkey is a single-stomached (monogastric) herbivore that eats rough-age, such as straw and hay, and is able to utilize cellulose and hemicellulose from plants very efficiently.[1] Donkeys are capable of digesting and processing low-quality feed as compared to horses. Their digestive systems adapted to arid areas with poor grazing, such as in Africa and Asia. Donkeys are termed "trickle feeders" and evolved to have fiber passing almost continuously through their gastrointestinal tract.[2] Consequently, when they are fed similar high-quality and high-calorie feeds as given to horses, they become over-weight and subject to nutritional-excess problems, such as obesity, laminitis, and hepatic (fatty liver) disease. Donkeys need more fiber and less protein in their diets than do horses. They are not ruminants so they must not be fed like cattle, sheep, or goats. Donkeys with access to cattle licks containing urea should be restricted in their intake to avoid urea poisoning.[3]

Feeding Behavior

Donkeys generally are more selective than horses in their food consumption, using their relatively narrow muzzles and mobile lips to sort through feed material. Like horses, they spend a great deal of time eating when turned out on pasture in favorable environmental conditions. Donkeys prefer shelter to rain and will remain inside when possible to avoid insects. They may search pastures for the most appealing plants if allowed free access to large areas, resulting in inefficient pasture use; rotational strip grazing is a more effi-cient method of pasture management. If feeding time is restricted in work-ing donkeys, they may resort to fast, incomplete chewing of forages, leading to digestive problems such as esophageal choke (obstruction) or intestinal impaction.[4]

Feeding Guidelines

- Allow all donkeys in a herd easy access to feed, regardless of age or activity level.
- An adequate quantity of clean, fresh water must be provided daily.
- Feeding time and method should be consistent to promote good digestion and to avoid problems.
- A working donkey should be allowed a rest period after a large meal. It is preferable to allow frequent, small meals throughout the day to simulate the normal feeding behavior of donkeys.
- Many donkeys will not eat or drink while in harness.[5]

Basic Nutritional Needs

The basic nutritional needs for all equines are: energy and calories (provided by dietary carbohydrates and fats), protein, water, and vitamins and minerals. Most often these needs may be met adequately through consumption of pasture plants and hay. The amount needed depends on climatic conditions and on individual metabolism. Donkeys in northern climates in the winter need more calories than in warmer months to offset the energy expenditure

3.1 A severely malnourished miniature donkey. Its legs are wrapped for treatment of pressure sores from lying on concrete floor.

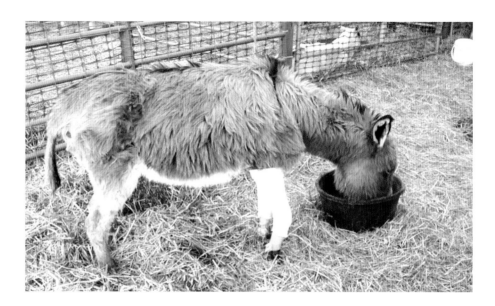

required to maintain body temperature. A limited amount of moderate quality hay and/or free choice, poorer quality pasture or hay may suffice for donkeys in warmer climates. It is important to regularly assess the body condition of each individual donkey to ensure that he is neither overweight nor too thin; the diet should be adjusted accordingly. It is equally important to ensure that all animals have equal access to food. If pastures are overgrazed due to over-crowding or if animals are kept in close proximity to larger or more aggressive animals, they will not be able to consume enough calories and may suffer serious weight loss or even die of starvation. This is especially critical for winter time feeding in northern climates.

The animal in fig. 3.1 was presented to a veterinarian in the early spring in the northeastern United States due to his inability to rise without assistance, the severe pressure sores on his legs, and his very poor body condition. Because of inclement weather, he had been kept inside where he had to compete with other horses and donkeys that were also in poor condition. His front legs were wrapped to protect the pressure sores caused by his being down on concrete flooring. The underlying problem was lack of sufficient food for all animals on the property. He survived and progressed to good health when this dietary management situation was corrected.

A study funded by the Donkey Sanctuary (www.thedonkeysanctuary.org.uk) and conducted by the University of Edinburgh and University of Central Mexico determined the maintenance requirements for fit, healthy donkeys. Results showed that donkeys require 1.3–1.7% of their body weight in forage daily, depending on the season; the lower value applies to summer. For maintenance, they needed 88–117 kJ DE (digestible energy)/kg of body weight), with the lower value corresponding to summer. In practical terms, this means that a donkey requires feedstuffs with low energy values so he can eat large enough quantities to satisfy his natural appetite without becoming obese.[6]

Energy Sources

Carbohydrates (CHO) are the primary source of calories for the donkey. They are exposed to pancreatic and intestinal enzymes before reaching their primary sites of fermentation in the cecum and colon. Starch, maltose, and sucrose are hydrolyzed and absorbed as monosaccharides (simple sugars) in the small intestine, proximal (forward) to the cecum. The primary sources of carbohydrates are forage crops: grasses (orchard grass, timothy, and brome) and legumes (alfalfa and clover). Legume hay or pasture is too high in protein and calories for donkeys and should be avoided. Common grains and horse feeds containing products like corn, oats, barley, wheat, and molasses should be avoided in donkeys.

Although the vast majority of donkeys can be fed adequately on a diet of straw along with limited hay and grazing, some animals require supplementary feeding due to advancing age or health problems. When devising a diet for these animals, it is important to satisfy the "trickle feeding" requirements of the donkey while taking into account underlying health problems such as poor dentition. It is important to avoid proprietary senior mixes or other energy-dense feeds (high fat or calories) as these not only oversupply energy but also do not provide the fiber component that is essential for the digestive health of the donkey.[7]

Energy requirements are increased as work level increases, as well as in late pregnancy, during lactation, during growth, or when exposed to low environmental temperatures. Adequate caloric intake is estimated by frequent assessment of body condition. To do this, donkeys should be palpated over the ribs, which should be able to be felt with minimal fat cushion, but should not be visible through the hair coat, especially in winter in cold climates.

Vitamins and Minerals

Minerals may be provided by free-choice, trace mineralized salt. They are also present in water to varying degrees and available in small amounts in forage and grain (if fed). Deficiencies of sodium and chloride are rare when there is adequate access to salt blocks.

There is debate regarding the need for supplemental feeding of vitamin E and selenium (Se) to donkeys. We know that in other species vitamin E functions as a cofactor with the cellular anti-oxidant, selenium. Plant sources of vitamin E deteriorate over time in stored hay. Some species of farm animals require selenium for maximum reproductive efficiency. Vitamin E is purported to help pregnant mares increase colostrum quality, milk production, and thus passive transfer of immunity (see p. 142) to their foals. Selenium is a cellular antioxidant and low selenium levels are implicated in the etiology of exercise-induced muscle damage (tying up syndrome) in horses. Vitamin E and selenium supplementation may play a role in prevention of reproductive abnormalities such as abortion, reduced fertility, early embryonic death, retained placenta, infertility, uterine infection, and birth of weak or premature horse foals.

Acid soils decrease available selenium from grasses. In general, it is important to know the relative selenium content of soils in the geographical area where your hay is grown as this then dictates if there is a need for selenium supplementation. Many horse breeding farms add supplemental vitamin E and Se to the ration of broodmares in geographical areas where it is deficient. However, there are no controlled studies suggesting that donkeys of any status require supplemental selenium in their diet. It is best to check with your local veterinarian.

Water

Fresh, clean water is an essential nutrient for donkeys to allow proper functioning of the digestive tract. Donkeys may refuse to drink dirty water or water with a taste different from what they are used to drinking. Donkeys have a lower water requirement than other domesticated animals, except the camel.[8] Environmental conditions and work level affect the volume of water that must be consumed. Donkeys can withstand up to 20 to 25% daily weight loss from dehydration yet can recover this loss quickly when water becomes available.[9] They are reported to be able to go without water for three days without harm when faced with severe water shortages.[10] However, when possible, it is not recommended to let any degree of dehydration occur. Also, donkeys should not be offered large amounts of very cold water when they are hot from working but should be allowed small sips as they cool off. Once cool, they should be allowed to drink their fill.

Hauling and Drinking

When being trailered, donkeys seem to prefer to face backward. Many owners transport them loose in a stock trailer rather than tying them in a confined area. Donkeys may not drink well when hauled or upon arrival at a new place, often going 12 to 18 hours without water. They can stay loaded on the trailer if a trip is less than 24 hours as long as stops are made every 4 to 6 hours to rest the animals. Water should be offered at rest stops. It is recommended to stop and unload every 12 hours if hauling more than 24 hours.[11]

Donkeys can dehydrate and lose 30% of body weight without adverse affects. They can also rehydrate quickly within 5 minutes of drinking.[3] They may refuse to drink for 48 to 96 hours if removed from their normal water supply. This may occur when hauling, showing, or if a donkey is hospitalized. It may be prudent to bring water from home and offer it in a familiar bucket when traveling. Keep in mind that some donkeys will not resume normal drinking and eating until after they have returned home.

Winter Feeding

Water consumption increases due to dry environmental conditions and the use of mainly dry food (hay and straw). Adding a sloppy, wheat bran mash to the diet at ½ pint to 1 quart daily (depending on body size) can add to water intake to assist gut motility. Donkeys need an ample daily source of clean, not frozen, water. Free choice hay should be provided when weather is extremely cold, but remain conscious of your donkey's body condition to avoid obesity. It is important to check body condition frequently to assess the adequacy of the diet. For some individuals, it may be difficult to gain weight during severe winter conditions, and for these donkeys, free-choice hay is appropriate.

Overfeeding

Overfeeding is one of the most common mistakes in managing donkeys. This leads to obesity (figs. 3.2 A–C) and associated risks of infertility, dystocia

3.2 A–C An obese jennet (A). Note the thick neck crest (1) and the fat deposits along the upper back (2). Excessive fat deposits evident in the crest (B) and over the gluteal region (C).

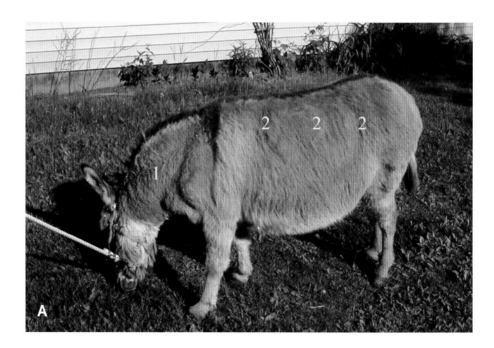

(difficult in foaling), and laminitis. Donkeys are particularly efficient feeders and easily become obese when allowed free access to high quality hay or pasture. Feeding of grain compounds the problem with the addition of even more calorie-dense foods. Donkeys will readily consume grains of all types, but grain should be restricted to underweight animals, late pregnant and lactating females, and growing foals less than one year of age if body condition warrants additional calories. Owners should carefully monitor the body condition of each individual and adjust caloric intake accordingly.

Feeding Obese Donkeys

Many donkeys kept as pets do little or no work and thus have relatively low caloric requirements. Donkeys usually always act hungry and can be quite insistent and vocal that they are "starving" for food, especially while other animals on the farm are being fed. Unknowing, but well-intentioned owners may respond incorrectly to this behavior by "giving a little grain once in a while"; over time this may result in a very obese animal. Obese donkeys need to have their caloric intake reduced, first and foremost. Good quality fiber is the basis of a healthy diet for donkeys. Grain supplementation must be ceased immediately to an obese animal. An owner must remain firm in resolve to correct the problem and to avoid serious health problems despite vocal behavior by

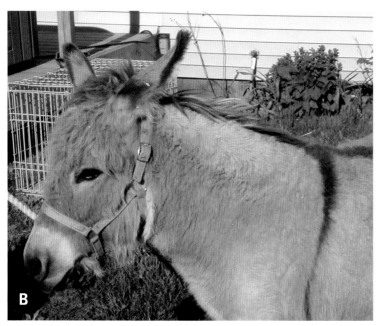
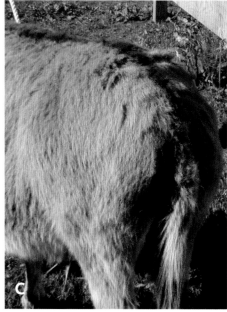

a donkey that is unhappy with reduced rations. Some methods of increasing caloric utilization to aid in weight loss include: walking, riding, and driving if appropriate, spreading feed over large areas to encourage walking at feed time, laying out strip grazing plots in pastures, and providing toys to prevent boredom and associated over-eating behavior.

Weight loss progress is often slow. The goal is to achieve progressive, gradual weight loss rather than a drastic, immediate drop in weight. The fat pads seen in obese donkeys in the rump, chest, and crest may not disappear even when an animal is returned to ideal body condition.

Malnutrition

Signs of dietary stress include poor hair coat, lack of energy, weight loss, and poor foot growth and body condition. These should be corrected by checking the quality and quantity of hay and pasture first, providing a mineral block, then only using supplemental grain as a last resort.

Sick animals may need special feeding to stimulate appetite. One of the following may be added to the hay for such a purpose: peppermint cordial, dried or fresh mint leaf, ginger, grated or chopped carrots, and apples.[12] Hand feeding or offering small quantities frequently may provoke interest in food since a sick donkey may be overwhelmed by the sight of a large bucket of feed. The natural instinct to browse may be used to advantage by taking a donkey to hedgerows or plant areas in the field to encourage eating.

Feeding old donkeys may be complicated by dental problems. These should be addressed and corrected as much as possible. It may be necessary to feed animals with bad teeth some type of chopped hay product or a softened mash made from complete feed pellets to aid in the first step of digestion.

Under-nutrition (see fig. 3.1, p. 18) may also be a problem especially when donkeys are turned out with full-size equines and competing for limited food. This depends on the temperament of the animals involved and the physical space allowed for access to food. Overcrowding often results in under-nutrition in the smaller or least aggressive animals and overfeeding of those at the top of the social order. These factors must not be overlooked. Owners should constantly evaluate the body condition of their animals and respond accordingly; this is especially important in the winter in cold climates.

Summary

- Donkeys may not drink well when traveling, hospitalized, or moved to new surroundings.

- Donkeys are capable of digesting and processing low-quality feed as compared to horses. Consequently, when they are fed similar high-quality and high-calorie feeds as given to horses, they become overweight and subject to nutritional-excess problems, such as obesity, laminitis, and hepatic (fatty liver) disease.

- A limited amount of moderate quality hay and/or free choice, poorer quality pasture or hay may suffice for donkeys in warmer climates. It is important to regularly assess the body condition of each individual donkey to ensure that he is neither overweight nor too thin; the diet should be adjusted accordingly.

- Fresh, clean water is an essential nutrient for donkeys to allow proper functioning of the digestive tract. Donkeys may refuse to drink dirty water or water with a taste different from what they are used to drinking. Donkeys have a lower water requirement than other domesticated animals, except the camel.[13]

- Overfeeding is one of the most common mistakes when managing donkeys. This leads to obesity and associated risks of infertility, dystocia, and laminitis. Donkeys are particularly efficient feeders and easily become obese when allowed free access to high quality hay or pasture.

- Signs of dietary stress include poor hair coat, lack of energy, weight loss, and poor foot growth and body condition. These should be corrected by checking the quality and quantity of hay and pasture first, providing a mineral block, and only using supplemental grain as a last resort.

- Under-nutrition may be a problem especially when donkeys are turned out with full-size equines and competing for limited food.

References

1. Aganga, AA; Letso, M; and Aganga, AO; Department of Animal Science and Production, Botswana College of Agriculture Gaborone, Botswana. "Feeding Donkeys." *Livestock Research for Rural Development.* 12(2), 2000.

2. Burden, F. The Donkey Sanctuary. "Donkey Clinical Welfare in Practice Meeting Proceedings." UK, October 2007.

3. See note 1 above.

4. See note 1 above.

5. See note 1 above.

6. See note 2 above.

7. See note 2 above.

8. See note 1 above.

9. See note 1 above.

10. See note 1 above.

11. Taylor, TS; Matthews, NS; Blanchard, TL. "Introduction to Donkeys in the US." *New England Journal of Large Animal Health.* 1(1): 21-28, 2001.

12. See note 2 above.

13. See note 1 above.

Herd Health

This section is an overview of the herd health procedures applicable to all donkeys. It includes information about deworming programs, nutrition, housing, vaccinations, and routine dentistry. Herd health for donkeys is similar to that for horses.

Equine vaccines and deworming medications may be used on donkeys with some restrictions although very little donkey-specific research has been performed in these areas. As discussed in chapter 3, overfeeding and subsequent obesity are common problems in donkeys. Routine dentistry is carried out in a similar fashion as for full-size equines, and it should be noted that bite abnormalities are relatively common in miniature equines.

Intestinal and Lungworm Parasite Control

Intestinal parasites affecting donkeys are similar to those that affect horses. These include nematodes (large and small strongyles, ascarids, and pinworms), bots, and cestodes (tapeworms). Basic principles of parasite control are the same as for larger equines. Medications used with success in donkeys include fenbendazole, ivermectin, albendazole, and pyrantel pamoate.

Animals in certain geographic locations are affected also by lungworms. These areas are not well defined. Donkeys are the natural hosts for lungworms and as such do not show obvious signs of disease when infected. In fact, the incidence of donkey infestation is not known. Mules are reported to be relatively unaffected by lungworm infestation, much like donkeys. Horses, however, may be severely affected, exhibiting coughing and wheezing. Lungworms should be suspected if an affected horse is pastured with donkeys or mules. Definitive diagnosis is made by demonstrating the presence of *Dictyocaulis arnfeldi* larvae in fresh feces. Treatment is achieved by oral dosing with ivermectin, followed by a repeat treatment in three weeks. (Lungworms are discussed in more detail in chapter 5, Infectious Respiratory Disease, p. 39.)

Other strategies of parasite control include pasture rotation, removal of manure, and deworming of new herd additions. Successful use or need for deworming medications should be measured by periodic fecal examinations. I recommend the sugar centrifugation technique of fecal analysis (see p. 39).

Vaccinations

Donkeys are vaccinated with the same products as full-size equines and with the same frequencies. However, there have been no conclusive studies regarding the effectiveness or safety of the equine products in donkeys. I was involved in a limited vaccination trial (unpublished study) with a small number of miniature donkeys. Titers were evaluated after vaccination with commercially available equine products against Eastern and Western encephalitis, equine herpes virus 1 and 4, equine influenza virus type A1 and A2, and Potomac horse fever (PHF). Results were inconclusive yet donkeys responded to these vaccines in the majority of instances as demonstrated by increasing titers, except for the PHF vaccine. (While only one brand of PHF vaccine was used, I still recommend vaccination against PHF in at-risk geographical locations.)

Some owners and veterinarians have suggested that miniature equines should be vaccinated with reduced doses of the standard equine vaccines. I do not recommend this practice as there is no scientific evidence for it and, in fact, the lower dose may not stimulate the immune system sufficiently to provide a protective response. No vaccine challenge studies have been or are likely to be performed in donkeys. Since 200-lb equine foals and 2,000-lb draft horses are given the same dose of vaccine, I recommend full-size, standard equine vaccine doses for donkeys of all sizes.

The specific vaccines used should be selected based on the disease risks in a particular location and the risk of infection from new arrivals and/or exposure at shows and events. This is particularly true for equine respiratory diseases. No data is available regarding the incidence of equine herpes virus abortion in donkeys therefore the practice of vaccinating donkeys at 5, 7, and 9 months of pregnancy has been questioned.

I have very limited experience with the use of vaccines against West Nile virus, and no experience with those for Venezuelan equine encephalitis and equine protozoal myelitis. An anecdotal report from one veterinarian in the northeastern United States revealed the West Nile virus vaccine to be non-reactive in miniature horses. Anecdotal reports from two miniature donkey owners in the Midwest revealed minimal side effects from the same vaccine. It is unlikely that any manufacturer will test effectiveness of any of these vaccines in donkeys. Their use should also be considered experimental from a safety perspective until more field use has been documented.

Feeding Practices

The basic necessities of clean, fresh water, trace mineral salt, and a source of dietary fiber and calories in the form of hay or pasture apply to donkeys. In full-size equines, a protein requirement of 8–10% may be safely applied. The specific nutritional requirements of donkeys have not been established. It is reasonable to apply horse data to donkeys, but the donkey's feral origin has adapted them to subsistence on low quality forages. (See chapter 3, p. 17, for a more detailed discussion.)

Dentistry

Routine dental care for donkeys is similar to that for horses. Small-sized dental floats are available for use in miniature donkeys. Bite abnormalities are relatively common in both miniature donkeys and miniature horses. This results from a lack of genetic diversity and reluctance of breeders to remove

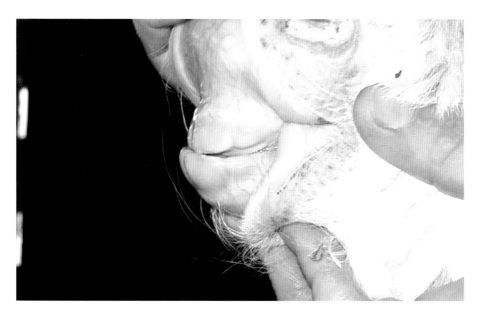

4.1 A juvenile miniature donkey with an under-bite. This disparity was present at birth but disappeared as the animal grew older.

animals with improper bites from their breeding programs. When size and sales become over-riding considerations, conformation often suffers. Both over and under-bites are common (fig. 4.1). These result in problems primarily with the incisor teeth, but severe abnormalities, may also affect the cheek teeth. Dwarfism is also relatively common in miniature equines, often accompanied by bite abnormalities, and a need for corrective dentistry is especially important in affected animals. Breeding decisions should be made with the long-term health of the animals as the major deciding factor. (See discussion in chapter 6, p. 70, for more detailed information on dentistry.)

Gastrointestinal Parasites

Major Intestinal Parasites

- Nematodes
  - Strongyles: large and small
  - Ascarids (roundworms)
  - Pinworms
- Cestodes (tapeworms)
- Bots (stomach worms)

Large and small strongyles are the most harmful of the equine intestinal parasites and equine deworming programs are aimed at control of these worms and their larvae. The large strongyle species (bloodworms) are approximately 1/2 inch long (1 cm) and reddish in color. The larval forms of these parasites may damage intestinal blood vessels and other organs during migration. Young animals are particularly susceptible to heavy infestations due to their immature immune system.

Large Strongyles

- *Strongylus equinus*: The buccal (mouth) cavity contains three teeth— one large and two small. Mature adult worms are 5 cm long.
- *Strongylus edentatus:* The buccal cavity is devoid of teeth. Mature adult worms are 4–5 cm long.
- *Strongylus vulgaris:* The buccal cavity contains two ear-shaped teeth. Mature adult worms are about 2 cm long.

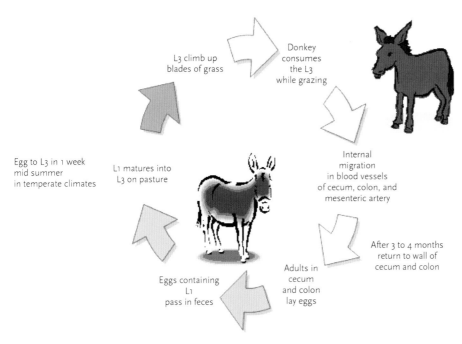

L3 climb up
blades of grass

Donkey
consumes
the L3
while grazing

Egg to L3 in 1 week
mid summer
in temperate climates

L1 matures into
L3 on pasture

Internal
migration
in blood vessels
of cecum, colon, and
mesenteric artery

After 3 to 4 months
return to wall of
cecum and colon

Eggs containing
L1
pass in feces

Adults in
cecum
and colon
lay eggs

The life cycles of all three large strongyles (fig. 4.2) have similar pre-infective phases. Adults are found in the cecum and colon of infected donkeys. Strongyle-type eggs are laid by mature female worms and pass to the environment in host feces. Hatching and larval development to an infective L3 (third stage larva) stage occurs within a temperature range of 8–38°C (50–100°F). Development from egg to L3 takes about 4–7 days in mid-summer in temperate climates. Infection is by ingestion of the ensheathed L3s when donkeys consume them with grass. After ingestion, the L3s penetrate the intestinal mucosa and molt to L4s within a week of ingestion. Then the L4s penetrate submucosal (beneath the intestinal lining) arteries and migrate along the endothelium (blood vessel wall lining) to the cecal and colic arteries (by 14 days post infection) and on to the root of the cranial mesenteric artery and its main branches by day 21 following infection. After a 3–4 month period of development, the larvae molt to immature adults (L5s), which then return to the intestinal wall via the arteries. Nodules form around the L5s mainly in the wall of the cecum and colon. Subsequent rupture of these nodules releases young adult parasites into the intestine where they mature in another 6–8 weeks. Adult male and females copulate and females lay eggs, which reach the external environment in host feces. The prepatent period (the interval between infection of a host and the earliest time at which eggs or larvae can be recovered from the host animal) for large strongyles is 6–7 months.[1]

Clinical signs of large strongyle infestation:

- Loss of condition
- Anemia
- Poor hair coat
- Diarrhea
- Colic
- Adult worms may be visible in droppings

Small Strongyles

Over 40 species of small strongyles (cyathostomes) have been found in the cecum and colon of domestic equines, each with its own site of preference. They belong to the subfamily *Cyathostominae* of the family *Strongylidae* and approximately 10 species are particularly prevalent. Most are appreciably smaller in size than the "large" strongyles.

The life cycle of the small strongyles is shown in fig. 4.3. Unlike the large strongyles, small strongyles do not migrate outside the intestine and early

4.3 The small strongyle life cycle.

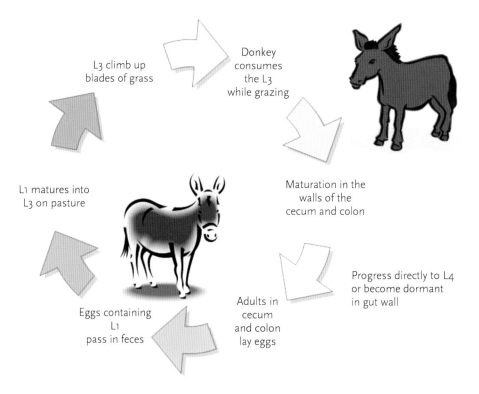

L3 climb up blades of grass

Donkey consumes the L3 while grazing

L1 matures into L3 on pasture

Maturation in the walls of the cecum and colon

Progress directly to L4 or become dormant in gut wall

Eggs containing L1 pass in feces

Adults in cecum and colon lay eggs

development is confined to the wall of the intestine. Third-stage larvae may progress to the fourth stage without interruption, or they may undergo hypobiosis (delayed development) to resume development after prolonged periods (months) of dormancy. When these worms emerge from the gut wall, they feed superficially on the mucosa and while this may rupture capillaries, they are less pathogenic than the large strongyles. Generally, the resulting erosions of the mucosa are hard to visualize.[2] Their damage comes from associated inflammatory responses in the intestinal wall.

Small strongyles may be implicated in an acute (sudden onset) syndrome of weight loss, often with severe diarrhea, seen more often in temperate areas in late winter and spring. This is associated with the mass emergence of previously hypobiotic larvae from the intestinal wall. Response to treatment is variable and prognosis for complete recovery may be difficult even with intensive therapy.[2]

Spread of Large and Small Strongyles

Eggs are passed in the feces and hatch into infective larvae in the environment. Larvae crawl up onto grass blades, particularly in moist conditions, and the donkey consumes the larvae during grazing. Over many months, these larvae mature within the donkey into an adult, egg-laying form. Infected donkeys contaminate the environment with eggs in the feces, and the cycle repeats.

Diagnosis of Large and Small Strongyle Infection

Fecal examination is the preferred method of diagnosis for strongyle infection. Note that small and large strongyle eggs have similar microscopic appearances. Centrifugation of feces in concentrated sugar solution (see p. 39) provides the best accuracy for diagnosis.

Roundworms

Parascaris equorum is the species name for the most common roundworm of donkeys. As adults, these worms can grow to 30 cm long, and if seen in feces, they appear stiff and white. They usually pose a problem in donkeys less than two years of age; young animals from 12 weeks to two years of age are most vulnerable. Roundworms do also infect older donkeys.

Life Cycle of Roundworms

The life cycle of *Parascaris equorum* is shown in fig. 4.4. The usual site of infection for roundworms is the small intestine. Eggs are passed in the feces of infected animals and at temperatures of 25–35°C (77–95°F), roundworm larvae become infective within 10 days. The infective stage is an egg containing a second stage larva (Egg+L2), which infects the donkey when ingested. These L2 larvae hatch in the gut and then migrate through the small intestinal wall to the liver. Most L2s reach the liver within 24 hours. Within 7–14 days following infection, the majority of larvae have migrated to the lungs through the heart and pulmonary arteries. L3s break out of the lung capillaries into the alveoli (air sacs) and migrate up the bronchial tree to the trachea and pharynx. Irritation there causes them to be coughed up and then swallowed. The final two parasitic molts (L3 to L4 to immature adults) take place in the small intestine. The prepatent period for ascarids ranges from 12–16 weeks, a much shorter interval than for strongyles.

4.4 *Parascaris equorum* life cycle.

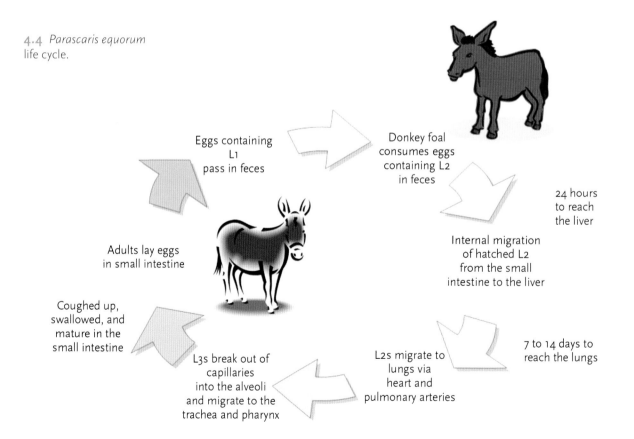

Eggs containing L1 pass in feces

Donkey foal consumes eggs containing L2 in feces

24 hours to reach the liver

Internal migration of hatched L2 from the small intestine to the liver

Adults lay eggs in small intestine

7 to 14 days to reach the lungs

Coughed up, swallowed, and mature in the small intestine

L3s break out of capillaries into the alveoli and migrate to the trachea and pharynx

L2s migrate to lungs via heart and pulmonary arteries

Clinical Signs and Diagnosis of Roundworm Infestation

In large numbers, roundworms may cause a loss of condition, diarrhea, or colic. In small numbers, they rarely cause any clinical signs. Roundworm infection is diagnosed by demonstration of eggs in fecal samples as for strongyles. The large, white adult worms may be seen in feces after deworming.

Pinworms (*Oxyuris equi*)

Adult pinworms are located in the large intestine and rectum, with female adults laying eggs around the anus. The irritation causes donkeys to back up to walls and trees to scratch and rub their rear end and anal region on these objects. Pinworms are diagnosed by microscopic examination of eggs on transparent tape samples taken around the anus.

Tapeworms

Three species of tapeworms are found in donkeys: *Anoplocephala magna*, *A. perfoliata*, and *Paranoplocephala mamillana*. They are 8–25 cm long (*A. magna* being the longest and *P. mamillana* the shortest). *A. magna* and *P. mamillana* usually localize in the small intestine but may also be found in the stomach. *A. perfoliata* is found mostly in the cecum but may also be found in the small intestine.

The tapeworm life cycle[3] (fig. 4.5) involves free-living oribatid soil mites as intermediate hosts. Tapeworm eggs are released by mature tapeworms that reside in the donkey's intestines; these eggs are passed in the feces. Mites typically break down organic matter and recycle environmental nutrients and also ingest tapeworm eggs found in the feces. These eggs mature within the mite to an immature stage of tapeworm. A grazing donkey inadvertently ingests infected mites as he forages, and once in a donkey's intestinal tract, the larval tapeworms attach to the donkey's intestines where they mature to an adult stage. Then, eggs are released once again to restart the cycle.

Clinical Signs and Diagnosis of Tapeworm Infection

With a light tapeworm infection, signs of disease are rarely present. In heavy infections, gastrointestinal (GI) disturbances may occur and unthriftiness and anemia may also be present. Intestinal perforation, peritonitis, and subsequent colic have been associated with *Anoplocephala* infections in horses.

4.5 The tapeworm
life cycle.

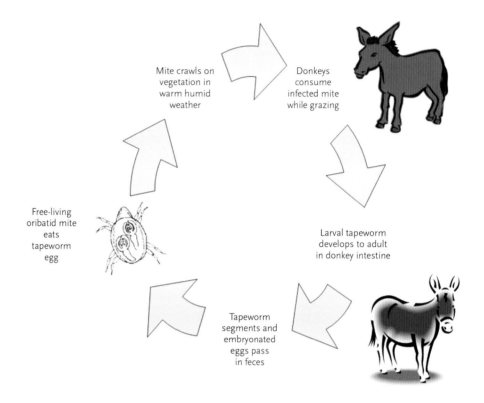

Mite crawls on
vegetation in
warm humid
weather

Donkeys
consume
infected mite
while grazing

Free-living
oribatid mite
eats
tapeworm
egg

Larval tapeworm
develops to adult
in donkey intestine

Tapeworm
segments and
embryonated
eggs pass
in feces

Donkeys that experience recurrent colic episodes should be dewormed for tapeworm infection even if eggs are not identified in the feces. There may be associated inflammation and ulceration at the attachment site of tapeworms and these injured areas may become infected.

An accurate diagnosis of tapeworm infection relies on demonstration of the characteristic eggs in the feces or finding worm segments in the manure. Because discharge of eggs and proglottids is sporadic, a single fecal examination may not be diagnostic. An ELISA (enzyme-linked immunosorbent assay) blood test is also available to evaluate for the presence of antibodies to tapeworm antigens (proteins), with varying results.

Bots

Strictly speaking, bots are not worms, but rather are insect larvae of equine bot flies. They are the most common parasite of the equine stomach. The life cycle of *Gasterophilus* species (bots) is shown in fig. 4.6. The small, white or yellow bot eggs are laid on the hair shafts of the donkey's legs and head. Female adult bot flies resemble bees and while laying eggs pose a considerable annoyance to the donkey. As a donkey rubs its legs with its face, hatched larvae enter the donkey's mouth and burrow into the base of the tongue and below the gum line. There, they double in size, and after a month, the bot larvae are swallowed and pass into the stomach where they attach to the stomach lining and continue development. If left untreated, bot larvae remain inside the donkey until the spring or early summer when they pass out in the manure. The larvae pupate underground with the adult flies emerging in middle to late summer to lay eggs, beginning the cycle anew. In a climate with distinct seasons, the first hard frost usually kills the adult flies and no re-infection occurs over the winter. Bots can affect donkeys of any age.

Bot larvae may give rise to ulcers in the stomach lining and chronic blood loss through bleeding. Potential penetration of the stomach wall could create peritonitis with possible fatal results, although this is an unusual occurrence. Bot larvae may also attach themselves in clumps to the uppermost portion of the small intestine, causing similar problems. This could pose a special danger for small breeds and to young donkeys whose stomach and intestines are likely to be thinner and more easily damaged.

4.6 The bot life cycle.

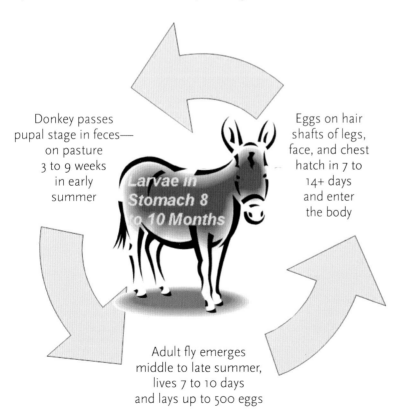

Donkey passes pupal stage in feces— on pasture 3 to 9 weeks in early summer

Larvae in Stomach 8 to 10 Months

Eggs on hair shafts of legs, face, and chest hatch in 7 to 14+ days and enter the body

Adult fly emerges middle to late summer, lives 7 to 10 days and lays up to 500 eggs

A presumptive diagnosis of bot infection is made by finding eggs on the hair shafts of the legs and head, particularly in summer and late fall. Some animals may rub their rear ends as bot larvae pass through the intestines in the manure in spring and early summer as part of the parasite's normal life cycle.

Diagnosis and Treatment of Intestinal Parasites

Prevention is the key to parasite control. Overcrowding and poor sanitation must be addressed to overcome parasite infestations, and to minimize the potential for reinfection. Parasite control programs should be designed for easy implementation. Reduction of the number of worms that are resistant to anthelmintic (anti-parasitic) drugs may be accomplished by selective deworming strategies based on the results of fecal examinations. It is thought that 20% of animals harbor 70–80% of the parasites. Strategies to reduce anti-parasitic drug resistance include: a) deworming only the animals in need based on serial fecal examinations, and b) by reducing the frequency with which they are dewormed. Effective parasite control strategies also rely on avoidance of sub-optimal nutrition, pasture contamination, and overstocking. (See fig. 4.7, p. 40, for comparative parasite egg sizes.)

Suggested Reading

• Carter, GR, and Payne, PA. *A Concise Guide to the Microbial and Parasitic Diseases of Horses*. International Veterinary Information Service, Ithaca, NY (www.ivis.org), 2007.
• Merck Veterinary Manual (www.merckvetmanual.com). Intestinal Diseases in Horses and Foals: Diarrheal Disease: Parasitism.

Deworming Programs

The goal of any deworming program is to interrupt the parasite life cycle. This may be done inside the donkey through the use of deworming medications. It is preferable to concentrate significant effort on management rather than relying heavily on medication. The parasite life cycle may be interrupted outside the donkey by frequent removal of manure, to limit the source of infection. Donkeys can also be moved off contaminated areas to minimize exposure to infective parasite stages. Pasture rotation is also effective in reducing pasture contamination. Alternating stocking of pastures with other livestock species, such as ruminants, allows non-equines to consume the parasitic larvae, which are not infective to them. Fecal exams should be performed on all new donkey arrivals to avoid contamination of pastures from stressed or heavily parasitized animals. New equine arrivals also should be isolated for three weeks before being turned out with the resident herd. Foals should not be exposed to transient animals, such as breeding animals, brought onto the farm.

Strategic deworming refers to deworming animals at specific times and under specific circumstances to increase effectiveness while minimizing use of drugs. Times when deworming might be appropriate include: a) before winter or frost; b) prior to going out on pasture; and c) tactical deworming 10–14 days after rain since wet conditions favor survival and development of infective parasite larvae. This will obviously not apply in locations that experience frequent rainfall. Effectiveness of dewormers should be checked periodically with fecal exams and deworming medications should be selected based on fecal counts of eggs per gram (EPG). A baseline fecal sample is analyzed just prior to administering an appropriate dosage of deworming medication and is then repeated 10–14 days later. If the EPG count does not decrease by at least 90%, then it is likely that resistance to the medication is occurring.

Parasite Diagnostic Procedure

The most accurate parasite examination technique involves using a concentrated sugar solution, which is mixed with the fecal sample. This solution is made by adding 2¾ cups of sugar to 1 pint of hot water and shaking vigorously until the sugar has dissolved. This solution's specific gravity is sufficient to float a high percentage of the parasite eggs to the top of the fluid layer when the sample is spun down in a centrifuge. The analysis procedure is as follows:

1 Wear gloves at all times when handling and processing donkey feces!

2 Collect fresh feces in plastic lock bag or plastic or rubber glove.

3 Mix one fecal ball with concentrated sugar.

4 Filter out large debris by pouring the mixture through a gauze pad or tea strainer.

5 Add the filtered mixture to a test tube.

6 Centrifuge for 10 minutes with a slide cover slip on in a swinging bucket centrifuge before viewing.

7 Or, centrifuge for 10 minutes in fixed rotor centrifuge, top off, add cover slip, and wait 10 more minutes.

8 Apply the cover slip to a microscope slide and view.

Microscope tips:

- Start by viewing slides on low power (10X objective and 10X eyepiece = 100X magnification).

- If having trouble finding the proper focus depth, move the stage so that the edge of the cover slip is directly under the lens (directly above the center of the light) and focus on that using the coarse and then fine focus knobs.

- Focus at the level of air bubbles—that is where the parasite eggs will be found.

- Adjust the light intensity so that you can easily see the slide without either being blinded or having to peer into darkness.

- Examine the entire area of the cover slip in a methodical pattern.

- Switch to 40X objective (total of 400X magnification) to focus on suspect parasite eggs after centering them in the visual field at low power.

- Don't get discouraged at first—everyone needs to practice to learn this.

4.7 Microscopic appearance of the eggs of the common intestinal parasites of donkeys showing relative size.

Roundworm

Tapeworm

Strongyle

Deworming Medications

Deworming medications are, in fact, poisons: they kill worms and worms are "animals" as are donkeys! Some drugs are excreted in active form in the feces and have harmful effects on the environment, killing beneficial creatures, such as dung beetles and earthworms. Dung beetles provide helpful effects like reducing the habitat that promotes development of nematode parasites and improving soil health, structure, and water infiltration of soil. They result in healthier pastures and increased pasture utilization by grazing livestock.

Equine deworming medications are divided into three main groups based on chemical composition (fig. 4.8):

- *Macrocyclic lactones:* ivermectins (Eqvalan® and Zimecterin®) and moxidectin (Quest®) (see below).

- *Benzimidazoles:* oxibendazole (Anthelcide®), fenbendazole (Panacur® and Safeguard®), and oxfendazole (Benzelmin®).

- *Pyrantel* (Strongid-P®, and Strongid-C® or Strongid-C-2X®)

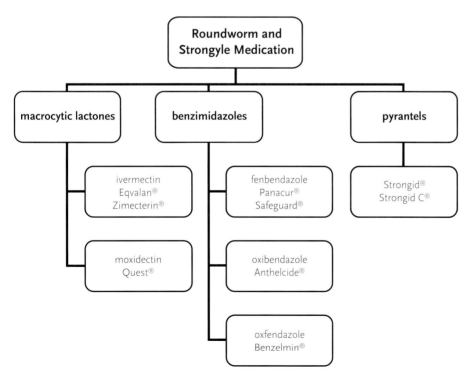

4.8 Medications commonly used to treat donkey intestinal parasites. Note that drug names are in lower case type while examples of product names are capitalized with the ® symbol after them. It is important to read the drug name on the package when deciding which medication to use as many products have the same ingredients although the name seems different.

Use of deworming products should be minimized with strategic protocols to protect beneficial soil inhabitants. Potentially problematic medications include ivermectin and moxidectin. In addition, moxidectin has a relatively low margin of safety and toxicity is seen at close to the therapeutic dose level. Overdosing a donkey with even a small amount could result in death. While many other deworming products are safe, there are no deworming medications approved specifically for use in donkeys.

There are various formulations of many brand name drugs such as oral liquids, pastes, and top dressings to put in feed. It is important to read the active ingredient on the label to ensure use of the appropriate and desired class of dewormer. Rotation of medication classes is considered by most to be the best strategy for drug use. Some believe that one medication should be used exclusively until resistance occurs but most veterinarians support a rotational medication scheme.

Medications successfully used to date to treat intestinal parasites in donkeys include:

- Large and small strongyles: benzimidazoles, macrocyclic lactones, pyrantel
- Encysted strongyles: fenbendazole given daily at double body weight dose for 5 consecutive days
- Roundworms: same as for strongyles
- Tapeworms: 2–3X body weight dose of pyrantel paste
- Bots: ivermectin
- Lungworms: ivermectin

So-called "natural," "holistic," or "new-wave" treatments against parasites include onions, garlic, and diatomaceous earth. To date, there are no controlled scientific studies proving their effectiveness or safety in any animal species.

Frequency of Dewormer Use

Overuse of dewormers may lead to more rapid development of drug resistant parasites. On the contrary, if medications are administered too infrequently, the ratio of parasite kill may be too low to ever get ahead of the infection, resulting in continual, internal damage to the animal and consequent malnourishment. An every-two-month frequency may be optimal to treat strongyles and roundworms in heavily populated or contaminated situations. It is recommended to treat 2–6 month old foals monthly with appropriate medications. Take special care of dosage if using medication with a narrow safety margin, such as moxidectin, so as to avoid adverse consequences.

Deworming frequency should also be determined by the parasite load of the individual donkey through periodic fecal egg counts (see p. 46). As a general rule, 20–25% of the herd, including poor doers and young animals, should be tested. Areas of high stocking density may necessitate frequent use of deworming medications in addition to diligent attention to pasture cleanliness and rotation. Parasite shedding is greatest in the spring and early summer, resulting in the heaviest pasture contamination at these times. Bot medication should be used following the first hard killing frost and after bot flies are gone. Likewise, tapeworm medication should be used seasonally when the mite intermediate hosts are no longer active in the soil.

Laboratory Tests and Reports

This section describes basic blood tests that may be performed to evaluate disease in donkeys. They are most often used to evaluate sick animals for evidence of infection or organ dysfunction with the goal of deciding treatment alternatives and prognosis. (See Appendix B, Donkey Reference Ranges for Blood Hemogram and Serum Chemistry Tests, p.150.)

Complete Blood Count (CBC)

The CBC evaluates the numbers and proportion of red and white blood cells. Blood is collected into a purple top tube with an anticoagulant so that individual cells may be counted and evaluated for appearance and type. If samples are not evaluated soon after collection, they should be preserved under refrigeration and evaluated within 24 hours if possible. Blood smears should also be made on the day of collection so that cellular appearances are not distorted or degraded with time. Blood smears should not be refrigerated to preserve the cellular architecture.

Red blood cell (RBC) tests include RBC count, hemoglobin, and hematocrit (HCT) also known as the packed cell volume (PCV). These parameters are used to evaluate animals for dehydration or anemia, and to measure if the animal is recovering from anemia, or not. An anemic animal has low RBC counts and low PCV. Dehydration means that the fluid component of the blood is lowered; the result is a relatively elevated PCV provided there has been no blood loss. As an example, in a case of colic, the degree of dehydration may be estimated to guide the amount of fluid replacement required with intravenous therapy. In contrast to the horse, severe dehydration does not commonly occur in the donkey.[4] Serial testing of PCV and total protein levels, along with monitoring of clinical signs, facilitate correction of dehydration. The degree of dehydration gives an estimate of the severity of circulatory compromise in sick animals. The higher the PCV, the worse the dehydration, and the more serious the disease process, with a poorer prognosis for recovery.

White blood cell (WBC) evaluation identifies the presence of infection or stress. Elevated white blood cell counts are typically associated with infectious processes yet also may occur when an animal is stressed. Overwhelming bacterial infections and some viral diseases result in a lowered white cell count. Serial WBC samples along with an improvement in attitude and appetite may be used to evaluate response to therapy.

A blood smear is used to evaluate the distribution of various types of white blood cells. There are established normal ranges for the white blood cell types (neutrophils, lymphocytes, monocytes, eosinophils, and basophils); alterations in their absolute numbers and relative proportions are associated with certain disease processes. For example, an elevated lymphocyte count is seen with a chronic infection whereas a recent bacterial infection typically results in an elevated neutrophil count.

Blood Chemistry Panel

Blood chemistry tests, also called serum chemistry, are used to evaluate organ function and protein levels in sick animals and to determine if animals that appear normal are suffering from organ dysfunction. Elevated serum protein levels indicate chronic infection or dehydration, while lowered levels indicate malnutrition, liver failure, or blood loss. Enzyme levels of liver, kidney, muscle, heart, and bone tissues are measured in the serum. Regular death and replacement of cells results in a relatively constant level of each enzyme within the bloodstream. If cellular injury or death occur at a higher than normal rate in a disease process, then organ function tests often demonstrate higher levels of "leakage" enzymes.

These chemistry tests require serum obtained by collecting the sample into a tube without an anticoagulant so that the blood clots. Samples should be refrigerated following collection and once the clot has formed, a centrifuge is used to spin clotted cells to the bottom of the tube, leaving the serum on top. Serum should be removed from the tube within 2–3 hours of collection to minimize artifactual abnormalities and to ensure accurate results.

The Coggins Test

Equine Infectious Anemia (EIA), also called swamp fever, is a viral infection of horses and donkeys. Historically, a blood test for the presence of antibodies to EIA has been called a "Coggins" test, which uses an agar gel immunodiffusion (AGID) method that is performed at federally approved laboratories. A positive test result indicates that the donkey is infected and serves as a carrier of the disease.

EIA virus is targeted in a national eradication program through testing; in addition, an equine isolation or euthanasia program has greatly reduced the incidence of the disease in the United States. This virus is spread from an infected equine through blood, such as in insect bites primarily from horseflies or deerflies, or from contaminated needles or equipment. Often, only one animal of a group may be affected even if all have the same exposure risk to bloodsucking insects. It takes approximately two weeks following infection for an animal to show positive for antibodies with testing, hence a negative test does not completely rule out infection. A negative test for EIA is always required for interstate and international travel of equines and is often requested for equine admittance to shows and events. It is recommended that a negative test result be a condition of sale when animals change owners.

Urinalysis

Urinary tract infections are not common in donkeys and neither is renal failure. However, microscopic and gross examination of the urine is undertaken to rule a disease problem in or out. A catheterized or midstream urine sample may be checked for the presence of abnormal protein or glucose levels, abnormal cells (blood or cancer cells), and specific gravity, which measures the ability of the kidneys to retain body fluid and concentrate the urine.

Fecal Examination

Feces may be examined for the presence of parasite eggs and/or larvae and protozoan oocysts. (These topics are covered in detail starting on p. 39.) Trace amounts of blood in manure may be invisible to the naked eye. Commercial fecal occult blood tests are available to check for this situation. A positive result may indicate the presence of a gastric or duodenal ulcer or another abnormality within the gastrointestinal tract, which requires further testing or medical treatment.

Microbial Cultures

Tissue and fluid samples, feces, milk, and uterine contents may be checked for the presence of bacteria, viruses, or fungi to identify the cause of infection. Bacterial culture and antibiotic sensitivity guides the use of relevant antibiotic therapy. A sterile swab is placed in contact with the tissue or fluid to be tested and then sealed in a container with transport media that provides bacterial nutrients during transfer to a laboratory for analysis. Special transport media that excludes air is necessary for anaerobic (only survive without oxygen) pathogens to survive until reaching the lab. The sample is then cultured under favorable growing conditions to allow any organisms present in the sample to flourish. The appearance, growth, and chemical reactions of the colonies growing on specialized media are used to identify the isolated organisms.

Antibiotic sensitivity disks are then applied to a culture plate covered with bacterial growth to check for kill zones that identify drugs useful in treating the infection. Sometimes, bacteria are sensitive or resistant to drugs within a laboratory setting (in vitro) yet will not display similar behavior in the live animal (in vivo). Other non-pathogenic or contaminant organisms must also be identified to avoid confusion with pathogens (disease-causing organisms). Aerobic bacteria (needing oxygen to survive) are identified commonly. Anaerobic bacteria may be found in some puncture or deep wounds, sinus infections, and some abscesses. If a fungus is suspected, as in a ringworm infection of the skin, specific fungal test media is necessary to facilitate growth; absence of fungal growth may require two to five weeks before being classified as negative.

Cytology

Cytology is the study of the structure and function of cells and is used to examine body fluids, such as abdominal and chest fluid, cerebrospinal fluid, joint fluid, urine, and uterine contents. Fluid from these locations is preserved in sterile tubes with anticoagulant for cytological examination and in bacterial culture tubes for bacterial identification. Cells from tumor masses are examined microscopically to determine the type of abnormal cells present to aid in choice of appropriate therapy. Some masses are, in fact, scar tissue and not neoplasia. A biopsy (acquisition of a piece of tissue) provides additional information when examined by a pathologist. Obtaining a tissue sample often requires chemical restraint with either sedation and local anesthesia or general anesthesia. A needle aspirate of a mass collects a very small sample of suspect tissue. It is the least invasive test but may lack accuracy if the sample is not representative of all underlying cell types. An incisional biopsy removes a piece of a mass, while an excisional biopsy removes all of the mass with all or part of it submitted to the lab, depending on its size. This allows the pathologist to make comments regarding whether the mass has been removed beyond the margins of the abnormal cells that may be present. Samples are submitted in a preservative such as formalin to maintain cellular architecture until a pathologist can process and examine thin sections microscopically.

Summary

- Routine herd health practices for donkeys of all sizes are similar to those for full-size horses with some exceptions as noted in this chapter.

- Equine vaccines and deworming medications may be used on donkeys with some restrictions although very little donkey-specific research has been performed in these areas.

- Routine dentistry is carried out in a similar fashion as for full-size equines, and it should be noted that bite abnormalities are relatively common in miniature donkeys and horses.

- More research needs to be performed in the areas of vaccination safety and effectiveness for donkeys.

- Sound breeding decisions are important to prevent conformational faults from adversely affecting the health of donkeys, just as in other breeds of livestock.

- The major intestinal parasites of the donkey are nematodes: large and small strongyles, ascarids (roundworms), and pinworms; cestodes (tapeworms); and bots (stomach worms).

- Large and small strongyles are the most harmful equine intestinal parasites and deworming programs are aimed at controlling these worms and their larvae.

- Clinical signs of parasite infestation include: loss of condition, anemia, poor hair coat, diarrhea, and colic.

- Prevention is the key to parasite control. Overcrowding and poor sanitation must be addressed to overcome parasite infestations, and to minimize the potential for reinfection.

- The goal of any deworming program is to interrupt the parasite life cycle. This may be done inside the donkey through the use of deworming medications. It is preferable to concentrate significant effort on management rather than relying heavily on medication. The parasite life cycle may be interrupted outside the donkey by frequent removal of manure, rotation of pastures, and alternating livestock species.

- Effectiveness of dewormers should be checked periodically with fecal exams, and deworming medications should be selected based on fecal counts of eggs per gram (EPG).

- The most accurate parasite examination technique involves using a concentrated sugar solution, which is mixed with the fecal sample.

- Use of deworming products should be minimized with strategic protocols to protect beneficial soil inhabitants. Potentially problematic medications include ivermectin and moxidectin. In addition, moxidectin has a relatively low margin of safety and toxicity is seen at close to the therapeutic dose level.

- Basic blood tests may be performed to evaluate disease in donkeys. They are most often used to evaluate sick animals for evidence of infection or organ dysfunction with the goal of deciding treatment alternatives and prognosis.

- Urinary tract infections are not common in donkeys and neither is renal failure. Microscopic and gross examination of the urine is undertaken to rule a disease problem in or out.

- Tissue and fluid samples, feces, milk, and uterine contents may be checked for the presence of bacteria, viruses, or fungi to identify the cause of infection.

- Cytology is the study of the structure and function of cells and is used to examine body fluids, such as abdominal and chest fluid, cerebrospinal fluid, joint fluid, urine, and uterine contents.

References

1. http://cal.vet.upenn.edu/projects/merial/index.html

2. Merck Veterinary Manual (www.merckvetmanual.com). Small strongyles: larval cyathostomiasis.

3. http://www.uky.edu/Ag/AnimalSciences/pubs/vet32.pdf

4. See note 1 above.

Infectious Diseases

Infectious Respiratory Disease

Infectious respiratory disease is a common problem in many animal species. In a survey of horse producers, respiratory disease was ranked as the most common medical problem of horses. A survey of veterinarians considered viral respiratory disease second only to colic in importance among medical problems of equines. Respiratory disease is equally important for the donkey. In addition, any respiratory condition, especially if accompanied by anorexia (lack of appetite), can precipitate life-threatening hyperlipemia (see p. 74) and gastric ulceration in donkeys. One British study suggested that anti-ulcer medication could be used for anorexic donkeys due to the high incidence of hyperlipemia and gastric ulcers found in postmortem exams of these donkeys.[1] The donkey is reported as having a different susceptibility to a number of diseases as compared to the horse, some of which are endemic (native to) throughout the world, e.g., African horse sickness, equine arteritis virus (EAV), equine infectious anemia (EIA) virus, and glanders.[2]

Viral and Bacterial Infections

Acute respiratory disease is known to be associated with several viral and bacterial pathogens. The viral agents most commonly associated with disease in donkeys are equine influenza virus and equine herpes virus. Another viral agent that commonly infects donkeys but is less commonly associated with clinical disease is equine arteritis virus (EAV). Bacterial pathogens may play a more important role as secondary invaders of donkeys infected with viral agents. In addition, *Streptococcus equi* is a common bacterial pathogen that causes primary respiratory disease. Clinical signs of respiratory disease are similar regardless of the agent involved and include: fever, mucopurulent (thick pus) nasal discharge, coughing, depression, and depressed appetite (inappetance). Coughing is less often seen with respiratory disease in donkeys than in horses.

Influenza virus is one of the more common contagious pathogens infecting equines throughout most of the world. In a number of experimental trials and natural outbreaks, the mortality has been higher and clinical signs more pronounced in the donkey than in horses.[3] Infected donkeys are more likely to develop secondary bacterial bronchopneumonia. Concurrent lungworm infection may also contribute to this higher mortality in donkeys.[4] I recommend that donkeys with respiratory infections be started right away on antibacterial drugs whether a virus is suspected as the cause or not, to prevent secondary bacterial infections. Epidemics may occur in groups of animals that are gathered for shows or athletic activity, or if a donkey incubating disease is brought onto a farm without implementation of routine biosecurity measures (see p. 60).

The incubation period from exposure to influenza virus to onset of clinical signs is 2–4 days. Clinical signs of influenza virus infection are a sudden onset of fever, nasal discharge, a characteristic dry cough, depression, and inappetance. An intermittent fever may be present for 2–5 days. Nasal discharge may be serous (thin and watery) early in the course of disease; it often becomes mucopurulent later when complicated by bacterial involvement. Animals with uncomplicated infections are reported to recover within 1–2 weeks of disease onset.

Suggested Reading

• Carter, GR, and Payne, PA. *A Concise Guide to the Microbial and Parasitic Diseases of Horses*. International Veterinary Information Service, Ithaca, NY (www.ivis.org), 2007.

Two types of equine herpes virus infection are commonly associated with respiratory disease in donkeys: equine herpes virus types 1 and 4, abbreviated as EHV-1 and EHV-4. Infections can be asymptomatic or cause only mild febrile (fever) episodes that are barely discernable. The incubation period is considered to be 2–10 days. Typical clinical signs associated with respiratory tract infections are seen, including serous nasal discharge that later becomes mucopurulent, anorexia, depression, mildly enlarged cranial and cervical lymph nodes, hyperemic (reddened) and congested nasal mucosa, and coughing.

Other diseases are caused by EHV: a) EHV-1 causes a paralytic neurologic disease and abortion in pregnant mares in addition to respiratory infection; b) EHV-4, in general, causes only respiratory disease. Neurologic disease caused by EHV-1 is rare. It is characterized by signs of ascending paresis (weakness) and paralysis, which are highly variable in severity. Clinical signs include: paraplegia (rear limb weakness), urinary and fecal incontinence, quadriplegia (weakness in front and rear), coma, and seizures.

EHV-1 is thought to be spread through direct or aerosolized contact with infectious material. The virus first infects the respiratory system, and then spreads to lymphoid tissues and leukocytes (white blood cells) of the peripheral blood, resulting in a cell-associated viremia (virus in the blood stream). Signs of respiratory disease are not always evident before abortion occurs or before the onset of neurologic disease. Latent (hidden) infections with EHV are an important feature that greatly affects the epidemiology of infection and disease caused in all host species. Latency is a type of persistent infection accompanied by intermittent episodes of shedding when a virus is reactivated months or years after the initial infection. Reoccurrence of EHV-1 and EHV-4 infection has been recognized in horses that have been isolated for many months with viral reemergence following stressful management events, such as weaning, surgical procedures, travel, or following administration of corticosteroid drugs.

Equine arteritis virus is an uncommon cause of respiratory disease in donkeys. It causes epidemics in horses, but subclinical infections are common. Clinical signs are variable and include serous or mucopurulent nasal discharge; occasional coughing; fever; conjunctivitis; edema (swelling) of the head, legs, prepuce (sheath), and abdomen; and abortion.

The bacterium *Streptococcus equi* is considered a primary pathogen in the equine species. A less pathogenic form, *Streptococcus zooepidemicus*, causes similar, yet less severe, clinical signs and is an opportunistic organism. The initial signs of disease include fever, depression, and inappetance. A mild cough and serous or mucopurulent nasal discharge may also be seen in early phases. The lymph nodes of the head and neck may become hot, swollen, and painful, which coincides with purulent lymphadenitis (swelling and inflammation of the lymph nodes), commonly referred to as "strangles."

Within a week of the onset of disease signs from *S. equi*, abscessed lymph nodes often rupture through the skin, or, in the case of abscessed retropharyngeal lymph nodes, into the guttural pouches (air-filled sac above the pharynx through which nerves and vessels run). Purulent nasal discharge and purulent drainage from abscesses can last for weeks after the initial malaise and depression have subsided. Signs of disease are highly variable and unexplained differences in clinical signs between infected animals might be attributable to differences in immunity to this organism. Respiratory disease cases infected with *S. equi* without showing evidence of lymphadenitis have been called "catarrhal" or "atypical" strangles cases, and these individuals serve as carriers of disease. "Bastard strangles" is the name for *S. equi* infections characterized by abscesses in areas other than the head and throat lymph nodes, such as lymph nodes in the hind legs or abdomen. Infection spreads to these locations through the lymphatic system.

Disease associated with *S. equi* is common in equines throughout the world and has been recognized for centuries. Auction barns seem to have a high incidence of strangles infections, which may spread to other facilities after transport.

Lungworms

Donkeys are the source of this respiratory-related nematode infection for horses although clinical disease in horses is uncommon. The lungworm *Dictyocaulus arnefieldi* (about 25–40 mm long) infects both horses and donkeys although patent (spreading) infections are usually only seen in donkeys and in foals; mature horses are more resistant. Adult lungworms live in the bronchioles, where females lay larvated eggs, which are coughed up, swallowed, and passed in the feces (fig. 5.1). The egg hatches within the feces before being passed out of the body. Development to the L3 or infective stage takes about 5 days on pasture.

After ingestion, the infective larvae migrate from the intestine via the lymphatics and the pulmonary arterial system to the bronchioles and bronchi where they mature. The prepatent period ranges from 6–8 weeks. Ordinarily, larvae do not develop into adults in the horse. Infections seem to be mild in the United States and less common in areas where broad spectrum anthelmintics have been used on a regular basis. In donkeys, and infrequently in foals, there is a persistent, moist cough and respiratory distress that may resemble signs of influenza. Diagnosis is obtained by finding first-stage larvae in feces using the Baerman fecal sedimentation procedure, although this is frequently unsuccessful. The finding of eosinophils in tracheal mucus has been used to support a diagnosis; however, finding mature lungworms at

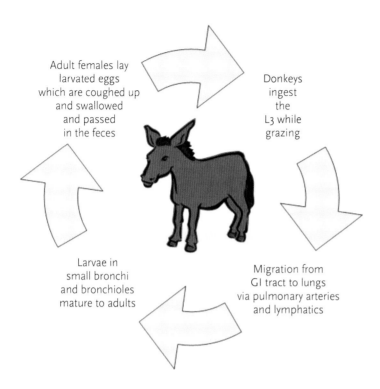

Adult females lay larvated eggs which are coughed up and swallowed and passed in the feces

Donkeys ingest the L3 while grazing

Larvae in small bronchi and bronchioles mature to adults

Migration from GI tract to lungs via pulmonary arteries and lymphatics

necropsy is the definitive diagnostic test. The avermectin class of drugs, such as ivermectin (see p. 38), is effective for treatment and control of lungworms in horses and donkeys.

Treatment

Basic treatment of respiratory infections in donkeys is similar to that for any species of animal. Common treatments include: rest; reduction of respiratory system irritants, such as dust and mold; isolation of sick donkeys; improved ventilation and fresh air; antibiotics involving anti-inflammatory drugs; cough medicines; and immune system stimulants.

Lungworm infections in donkeys are treated by a single dose of oral ivermectin (200 µg/kg body weight). Recently, oral moxidectin (0.4 mg/kg) has been shown to have efficacy against lungworms. This parasite can be hard to eliminate from paddocks due to prolonged survival in cool, moist conditions. Pasture management—harrowing, plowing, or rotation—may reduce numbers of larvae, and larvae do not survive severe frost. Once eradicated from the environment, the long prepatent period of lungworm means reinfestation is slow, especially if ivermectin or moxidectin is being use as an anthelmintic to control intestinal nematodes.[5]

Diarrhea in Donkeys

Diarrhea is defined as an increased frequency and discharge of abnormally watery feces. It results in water and important electrolyte (salt) loss greater than that taken in; this leads to imbalances with potentially severe consequences (fig. 5.2).

Mechanism and Results

Two main forms of diarrhea exist: hypersecretion and malabsorption. Roughly 25% of body water normally cycles through the intestinal tract daily. In a case of hypersecretion-type diarrhea, as seen with the bacteria *Escherichia coli (E. coli)*, water is secreted into the intestine in excess of normal fluid reabsorption in the GI tract. In malabsorption-type diarrhea, as occurs with most other intestinal infectious agents, there is normal fluid secretion into the intestine, but reduced transfer (malabsorption) from the bowel back into the circulation.

Diarrhea results in body fluid loss; if severe enough, it also leads to clinical dehydration. Dehydration is evidenced by dryness in the mouth and reduced temperature in the lower limbs and ears due to impaired circulation resulting from fluid loss. The eyes may appear to sink in the eye sockets with a gap appearing between the eyeball and inner lid. If dehydration is severe enough, urine output declines with possible kidney failure. Body electrolyte losses and imbalances also affect heart and skeletal muscle function.

It is important to detect diarrheic animals to determine the underlying cause and to implement fluid and electrolyte replacement before losses become too profound.

Causes

Irritation and inflammation of the intestinal mucosa (lining) due to infectious microorganisms or parasites results in malabsorption of fluid, electrolytes, and nutrients. This may also result in increased gut peristalsis (contractions) pushing contents through the intestines more quickly than the normal absorption and digestion processes can be completed. Poor digestion may alter the normal microflora (bacteria, fungi, viruses, and protozoa) necessary for proper digestive function. Dietary changes, particularly if rapid, may cause an overgrowth of pathogenic bacteria.

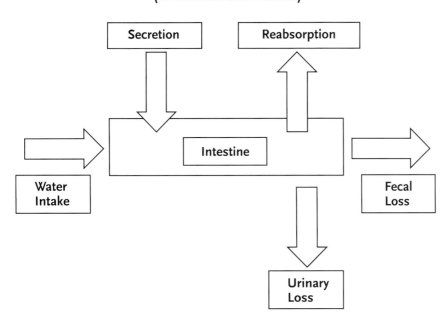

**Body Fluids
(Circulation and Tissues)**

Secretion

Reabsorption

Intestine

Water
Intake

Fecal
Loss

Urinary
Loss

Acute diarrhea in adult donkeys is caused by: a) bacteria such as *Salmonella* and *Clostridium spp*; b) viral infections; c) poisonous plants such as oak (acorns, blossoms, buds, and leaves); d) chemical causes such as arsenic, mercury, linseed oil, organophosphate insecticides, salt, and selenium; e) mycotoxins (toxins produced by molds); f) consumption of a large quantity of grain, which may also cause colic or laminitis; g) the sudden introduction of pasture or grain into the diet.

It is reasonable to assume that the causes of diarrhea in donkey foals are similar to the causes of diarrhea in horse foals although very little is published on this subject. The horse foal is affected by bacteria such as *Salmonella* and *Clostridium perfringens* type C, and viruses such as *Coronavirus*, *Adenovirus*, *Rotavirus*, and *Equine Herpes virus* 1. Antibiotics such as erythromycin and protozoa such as *Cryptosporidium* or *Coccidia sp.* also may cause acute onset diarrhea in horse foals. Nutritional causes of diarrhea in foals include: overfeeding milk replacer; nursing on high lactating jennets; changes in diet; and ingestion of sand, dirt, weeds or toxic plants. Infectious diarrhea in foals is often accompanied by fever and depression. Foal heat scours is reported to occur in 75–80% of horse foals in conjunction with the mare's first heat cycle following foaling. The stress of separating a foal from his mother can also induce diarrhea. Parasites such as *Strongyloides* that are passed through the mare's milk, any change in the composition of the mother's milk, and physiological changes in the foal's GI tract as normal bacterial flora develop are possible other reasons for diarrhea in foals.

Chronic diarrhea is defined as diarrhea that persists for at least 7–14 days or recurs after a period of remission. Associated clinical signs include persistent or intermittent diarrhea of variable consistency (watery to cow-pie), fever, lack of appetite, depression, weight loss, and chronic or recurrent colic. Subcutaneous (beneath the skin) edema may be seen in the sheath, lower abdominal wall, or lower limbs if excessive amounts of protein are lost through the feces or if it is not absorbed normally from the bowel. A normal level of blood protein is necessary to maintain the correct amount of water in the blood stream. If protein levels decline too far, then fluid leaks from blood vessels to accumulate in the soft tissues, with resulting edema. Causes of chronic diarrhea include: intestinal parasites, cancer (intestinal lymphosarcoma), inflammatory bowel disease, nonsteroidal anti-inflammatory drug toxicity (in horses), *Salmonella* infection, chronic liver disease, and sand irritation to the bowel.

Diagnosis

In attempting to isolate a cause of diarrhea, it is helpful to perform a fecal exam to look for parasite eggs, protozoa, sand or gravel, or blood. A fecal culture may be useful to identify a bacterial infection, as for example *Salmonella*. Depending on the severity and chronicity of the diarrhea, it may be prudent to run a CBC and chemistry panel. The basic physical exam is, of course, always performed on any equine with diarrhea or showing signs of sickness. Management and dietary history help to identify potential dietary causes. Rectal examination may reveal abnormal GI tract contents or tumor masses while an abdominal ultrasound exam and/or radiograph may reveal the presence of sand in the lowest sections of bowel where sand is most likely to accumulate.

Treatment

The exact treatment of diarrhea in donkeys depends on the actual or probable cause of the problem. Foal heat scours may be treated with oral administration of bismuth subsalicylate (e.g. Pepto-Bismol™ at a dose of 60 cc per 100 lbs body weight, 3–4 times daily) until the stool firms up. While large volumes are needed for an adult, this medicine should be used with caution in foals to avoid creating constipation. Symptomatic treatment may consist of a few days of daily treatment with an oral probiotic paste or powder, or with yogurt. If a bacterial infection is suspected, then antibiotic therapy may be indicated under advisement from your veterinarian. A viral infection is not responsive to antibiotic therapy so antibiotics would only be used if there is evidence or concern that the donkey has contracted a pathogenic bacterial infection, as well. Antibiotics may also be used to prevent potentially life-threatening secondary bacterial infections in cases where specific diagnoses are not undertaken, nor possible.

If high numbers of parasite eggs are found on fecal exam, then larvicidal doses of anthelmintics, such as ivermectin or fenbendazole, may be administered if the donkey is not in too compromised a physical state. Sand accumulation is treated by administration of oral psyllium per label directions. Nutritional support may be necessary to correct protein and electrolyte losses. This may consist of high-protein hay and/or grain, vitamins, and minerals as prescribed by your veterinarian. Eliminating lush grass and grain from the diet improves ease of digestibility of feed.

Oral or intravenous fluid therapy may be indicated depending on the degree of dehydration in individual cases. Useful guidelines for treating dehydration apply to many animal species, the donkey included. An animal with fluid losses of less than 5% of total body weight is generally still standing, the eyes are bright, the oral mucous membranes are moist, and tenting of the skin when pinched over a bony prominence such as the upper eye socket returns to normal within 2–4 seconds. Foals continue to nurse if dehydration is mild. Mildly dehydrated animals can be treated with an electrolyte mix in water that is offered in a bucket or by oral dosing.

Moderate fluid loss of approximately 7% of normal body weight creates a state of dehydration characterized by a dull attitude and posture; a foal may lie down in a sternal position. With moderate dehydration, donkey skin "tents" for at least 5 seconds, the eyes are sunken slightly, the limbs feel cold to the touch, and the oral mucus membranes are somewhat tacky. Such an affected animal needs warm, high-energy electrolyte solutions given by stomach tube and also by the intravenous route. Glucose included in the replacement therapy provides energy to promote fluid absorption and for nutrition. An animal in this compromised state, especially if a foal, should also be moved to a warm area where it can be monitored closely.

With severe fluid losses of more than 8% of body weight, the animal is often lying flat, and may be non-responsive to stimuli or in a coma. The skin remains "tented" when pinched, the eyes are deeply sunken, the limbs and face feel cold, and oral mucous membranes are cold, pale, and dry to the touch. Intravenous fluids are imperative to attempt to save these animals because oral fluids will not be absorbed sufficiently by inadequate systemic circulation. An animal in this state is best cared for at a veterinary clinic and should be transported there immediately.[6]

Diarrhea Problems Seen in Clinical Practice

- Associated with change of diet: treat by returning to original diet and possibly supplementing with probiotics or yogurt.

- Parasitic diarrhea: responds to anthelmintic medications.

- Infectious diarrhea: treat with antibiotics when indicated; fluids (oral and/or intravenous); management of endotoxemia; prophylactic prevention of laminitis; may also benefit from use of probiotics.

Note that *Salmonella* bacteria and the protozoa *Cryptosporidium* are highly contagious to humans. Whenever an outbreak of diarrhea occurs on a farm, it should be considered that a disease entity is present that may affect humans and other livestock on the property. Appropriate biosecurity measures should be implemented immediately.

Biosecurity for Donkey Farms

Biosecurity is defined as "security from transmission of infectious diseases, parasites, and pests" (*Saunders' Comprehensive Veterinary Dictionary*, 2nd edition, 1999). The goal of a biosecurity program is to prevent the introduction of new diseases and to control or eradicate disease that has entered the farm.

Disease Control

Diseases enter a herd from a variety of sources including: environmental contamination (feces, bedding, feed, water, wheelbarrows, rakes, and animals, such as rodents, birds, insects, deer, and dogs); new equine additions to the herd; visitors carrying disease agents from other farms on their clothing or shoes; animals coming in for breeding or returning from breeding farms; and by animals returning from shows. A farm manager's task is to minimize or eliminate these sources of infection.

Transmission of Disease

When an animal is exposed to a disease agent, several results are possible:

- The animal may be affected by acute, clinical disease, and be obviously sick. An infected animal may shed infectious particles after exposure and be a source of infection for others.

- The animal may be incubating an infectious agent yet show no clinical signs. As a carrier, the animal may not be sick but can spread the disease to other animals.

- An exposed animal may eliminate disease agents without developing illness, without shedding, or may not establish a carrier state.

The reaction of individual members in the herd also depends on the specific disease agent involved. Some agents are more virulent than others and are more likely to result in infection and clinical disease. The amount and duration of exposure to the infectious agent is another important factor to be considered. The immune status of each animal determines whether an exposed animal contracts an infection or not. The age of the animals exposed is another risk factor as younger animals have immature immune systems and are more susceptible to infections. Genetics also plays a role in that some families have better disease resistance than others. The presence of concurrent disease such as parasites and malnutrition additionally affects an animal's ability to resist disease.

Spread of Disease

Diseases are spread by a variety of means, such as: physical contact with other animals including humans; body fluids; respiratory secretions; urine; uterine fluids; diseased tissues (e.g. placenta); feces; insects; fomites (inanimate objects); and environmental contact with disease organisms.

A disease spread by physical contact can be transmitted from fluid contained in blisters as seen with Vesicular Stomatitis virus, from skin contact with a fungus like ringworm, or through external parasites, such as lice and mange. Fecal contamination with pathogenic strains of *Salmonella*, *E. coli*, *Rotavirus*, or internal parasites and protozoa may transmit infection. Fomites, such as water buckets and tanks; feeders; stall walls and aisles; clothing or hands of handlers; visitors; veterinarians and grooms; and trailers and other vehicles are able to pass disease organisms, particularly respiratory bacteria or viruses, to animals. Used needles and equipment can pass blood materials and potential infection.

Diseases spread between species include rabies (via saliva in a bite from an infected mammal); *Salmonella* (birds, mammals, and reptiles); Vesicular Stomatitis virus (sheep, pigs, cattle, and horses); intestinal nematodes (horses); and *Cryptosporidium* and *Giardia* (many species). Fecal spread of disease is significant with intestinal parasites, bacteria (*Salmonella*), protozoa (coccidia, *Cryptosporidium*, and *Giardia*), and viruses (*Rotavirus*, *Coronavirus*). Diseases spread by insects to donkeys include West Nile virus and Eastern equine encephalitis (via mosquitoes from birds); Lyme disease (via ticks from deer); Equine Infectious Anemia virus (via large biting flies); and tapeworms (via soil mites). Environmental diseases of significance to donkeys include tetanus from spores in the soil; rain rot (the bacteria *Dermatophilis congolensi*, a soil organism); and intestinal parasites via oral exposure to contaminated ground, feed, water, or pasture.

Isolation or quarantine facilities are useful to prevent the spread of disease from newly arrived animals. Isolation of a new arrival allows observation for signs of disease while allowing time to achieve results from diagnostic tests before a new arrival is allowed to comingle with the resident herd. Ideally, an isolation arrangement should be implemented for 3–4 weeks, with physical separation of at least 150 feet away from other animals and no possibility of physical contact or contamination by feces or urine. Caretakers should have limited contact with the new animals while isolated animals should be handled last with handlers wearing shoes and clothing dedicated only to their care.

Pre-Arrival Testing for New Additions to the Herd

Tests in advance of introducing a new donkey to the farm will help prevent introduction of disease. A physical examination for overt clinical disease should be performed at the farm of origin. It is always good practice to require that an animal be accompanied by a recent certificate of veterinary examination (health inspection) and a negative Coggins test prior to being admitted onto your property.

Laboratory tests prior to transport should include testing for Equine Infectious Anemia (EIA) virus (see Coggins test, p. 45) and fecal testing for intestinal parasites (see p. 46). USDA (United States Department of Agriculture) interstate travel regulations require EIA testing to cross state borders, and international travel requires thorough testing for a variety of other diseases in addition to EIA, the specifics of which are determined by the country to which the donkey will travel. Each state has its own required testing and timing of the Coggins test for entry—some require a test within 6 months while others only require it within a year. An interstate or international health certificate must be completed by a licensed and federally accredited veterinarian; timing of the health exam prior to admittance into different states or countries varies according to their specified rules. Some states also require an entry permit and number that are issued by the receiving state prior to entry of an animal. Interstate travel requirements for the United States may be found at www.aphis.usda.gov.

Post-Arrival Procedures for New Additions to the Herd

Once an animal has been admitted to the farm, it should receive a thorough exam to identify problems, such as diarrhea, lack of appetite, fever, coughing, ocular or nasal discharge, elevated respiratory rate, poor body condition, and skin abnormalities. A fecal exam for intestinal parasites is recommended upon arrival, as well, and treatment should be initiated based on the results. It may be appropriate to retest and retreat some individuals with a heavy parasite load. New additions to the herd should be physically isolated from the resident farm population for about 3–4 weeks, with particular care taken to keep new arrivals away from foals and pregnant animals.

Females and studs visiting for breeding should be quarantined entirely away from the resident herd. All breeding activities are best conducted in a location separate from the rest of the herd. Behavior testing for the presence of estrus may be accomplished using a resident jack to avoid exposing a breeding jennet to additional animals outside her resident herd. Farm staff should practice strict sanitary precautions to prevent introduction of disease into the resident farm population or to the quarantined animals. Human visitors should not be allowed near quarantined animals. Non-composted manure from quarantined animals should not be spread on pastures and quarantine facilities should be disinfected before repopulation.

Biosecurity for Show Animals

Shows are high-risk situations that mix many animals from various different locations and management conditions. Animals are often stressed at shows, which weakens the immune system and increases the chance of contracting disease or the shedding of infectious organisms by carriers. Common diseases that develop at shows or shortly after are often associated with respiratory tract infections. These are not likely to occur at shows of one-to-two-days duration but may become obvious at longer shows or after the show animals return home.

Show animals should be isolated from the resident herd when they return home, with strong consideration for having a separate barn dedicated to them during the traveling season. During the show, do not allow your animals to contact those from other farms. This may necessitate putting up barriers between your animals and those in adjacent pens. Position your donkey as much as possible to achieve physical separation in the waiting area adjacent to the show ring. Avoid allowing your animals to "visit" other animals on the show grounds. Refrain from walking your animals through the show facilities or grazing on grass or hay where other animals are standing or eliminating wastes. Stricter biosecurity measures are also possible to minimize infection risk, such as providing disinfectant hand wipes for visitors to use before and after they touch your animals, as well as locating disinfectant foot mats at stall entrances.

Protecting Your Herd

Prevention is the key to avoiding infectious disease transmission. Use of vaccinations improves the immune system status of your herd. Full protection from influenza and rhinopneumonitis vaccines may persist for only 3 months, depending on the product used. Use these vaccines around the time your animals will be exposed to high-risk situations, like a show or event. Ideally, booster your donkey at least 10–14 days before an anticipated risk. The selection of vaccines should be based upon advice of local veterinarians.

Good nutrition is also essential to producing a competent immune system and maximal resistance to disease. To minimize herd stress, allow your donkeys to form small social groups based on compatible temperament, body size and condition. Keep pastures, barns, and water sources clean, and limit animal access to ponds, streams, swamps, and muddy areas.

Insect control is important to prevent insect-transmitted diseases such as Eastern equine encephalitis and West Nile virus. Try to avoid turnout during active mosquito feeding times. Use safe insect repellants or traps and eliminate sources of stagnant water where mosquitoes breed.

Disinfectants

Many chemical disinfectants inactivate viruses and bacteria. For optimal use, it is necessary to brush and scrub away dirt, manure, and debris before applying disinfectant. Spray or dip shoes in a disinfectant foot bath or provide disposable shoe covers for all farm visitors. Some useful disinfectants include chlorine bleach (¾ cup per gallon of water or 1 part bleach to 10 parts water); One Stroke Environ® (Steris Corporation); and Tek-trol® (Bio-Tek Industries). The last two products are effective for foot baths and cleaning of floor mats, stall walls, and trailers.

Summary

- Infectious respiratory disease is a common problem in equines including the donkey. Any respiratory condition, especially if accompanied by anorexia (lack of appetite), can precipitate life-threatening hyperlipemia and gastric ulceration in donkeys.

- Acute respiratory disease is known to be associated with several viral and bacterial pathogens including equine influenza virus, equine herpes virus, equine arteritis virus, and *Streptococcus equi* and *zooepidemicus*.

- Donkeys are the source of the respiratory-related lungworm nematode infection for horses although clinical disease in horses is uncommon. In donkeys, and infrequently in foals, there is a persistent, moist cough and respiratory distress that may resemble signs of influenza.

- Diarrhea is defined as an increased frequency and discharge of abnormally watery feces. It results in water and important electrolyte (salt) loss greater than that taken in; this leads to imbalances with potentially severe consequences.

* It is important to detect diarrheic animals to determine the underlying cause and to implement fluid and electrolyte replacement before losses become too profound.

* Irritation and inflammation of the intestinal mucosa (lining) due to infectious microorganisms or parasites results in malabsorption of fluid, electrolytes, and nutrients.

* Acute diarrhea in adult donkeys is caused by bacteria, viral infections, poisonous plants, chemical causes, mycotoxins, consumption of a large quantity of grain, or the sudden introduction of pasture or grain into the diet.

* It is reasonable to assume that the causes of diarrhea in donkey foals are similar to the causes of diarrhea in horse foals although very little is published on this subject.

* Causes of chronic diarrhea include: intestinal parasites, cancer, inflammatory bowel disease, nonsteroidal anti-inflammatory drug toxicity (in horses), *Salmonella* infection, chronic liver disease, and sand irritation to the bowel.

* Determination of the possible cause of diarrhea may include: performance of a fecal exam, a fecal culture, a CBC and chemistry panel, a basic physical exam, review of management and dietary history, rectal examination, and abdominal ultrasound exam and/or radiography.

* The exact treatment of diarrhea in donkeys depends on the actual or probable cause of the problem. Possible treatments include: bismuth subsalicylate, antibiotics, probiotics, oral or intravenous fluids, and anthelmintics.

* The goal of a biosecurity program is to prevent the introduction of new diseases and to control or eradicate disease that has entered the farm.

* When an animal is exposed to a disease agent, several results are possible: acute, clinical disease, shedding infectious particles after exposure and serving as a source of infection for others, establishment of a carrier state, or elimination of the disease agent without developing illness.

- The reaction of individual members in the herd also depends on the specific disease agent involved, the amount and duration of exposure to the infectious agent, the immune status of each animal, the age of the animals exposed, genetics, and the presence of concurrent disease.

- Diseases are spread by a variety of means, such as: physical contact with other animals including humans; body fluids; respiratory secretions; urine; uterine fluids; diseased tissues (e.g. placenta); feces; insects; fomites (inanimate objects); and environmental contact with disease organisms.

- Pre-arrival testing and post-arrival procedures for new additions to the herd will help prevent introduction of disease.

- Shows are high-risk situations that mix many animals from various different locations and management conditions.

- Prevention is the key to avoiding infectious disease transmission. Use of vaccinations, minimizing stress, insect control, and use of disinfectants and quarantine procedures are important to achieve this goal.

References

1. Thieman, AK, and Bell, NJ. "The Peculiarities of Donkey Respiratory Disease." International Veterinary Information Service (www.ivis.org), Equine Respiratory Disease, 2001.

2. See note 1 above.

3. See note 1 above.

4. See note 1 above.

5. See note 1 above.

6. Yousef, MK; Dill, DB; Mayes, MG. "Shifts in body fluids during dehydration in the burro, *Equus asinus.*" *Journal of Applied Physiology.* 1970; 29:345-349.

The Digestive System

The Digestive Tract

The anatomy of the donkey digestive system is similar to that of the horse. The major components work in unison to make donkeys very efficient converters of consumed forage even if it is low in digestible quality or nutritional composition. Digestive tract components include the mouth, esophagus, stomach, small intestine, large intestine (cecum and colon), and the rectum. The term gastrointestinal tract (GI tract) is used to describe the components starting at the stomach and ending downstream with the rectum.

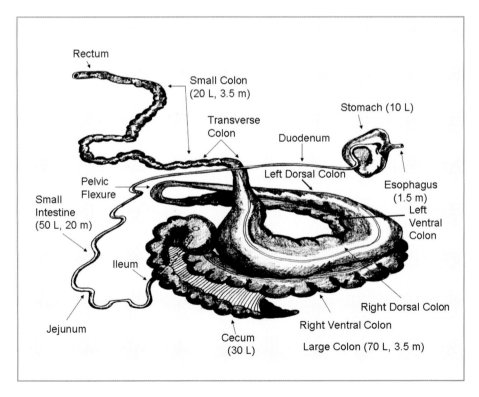

6.1 A diagrammatic representation of the donkey's gastrointestinal (GI) tract. Measurements noted are for 1,000 lb horses and are approximate for the same size donkey.

Mouth

A donkey's lips are very sensitive and flexible. They allow careful selection of plants to grab with the teeth and start the digestive process. Donkeys rarely eat foreign objects even if grazing in areas with garbage. Teeth break the food into small pieces, which can be easily swallowed. Donkeys chew their food carefully so that when it reaches the stomach it is in the proper shape and size to be acted upon by stomach acid. Chewing adds saliva to the food allowing for easier breakdown and swallowing. Drier food requires longer chewing time and necessitates production of more saliva. Donkeys are not prone to esophageal obstruction (choke) from swallowing large amounts of food at once; however, choke may occur if an animal is a greedy eater, has been restricted from food for a long time, or if he rapidly consumes pelleted feed, which may swell and become trapped in the esophagus.[1]

Teeth

The deciduous (temporary or baby) teeth of a young donkey are replaced by the permanent teeth between the ages of 2½ and 4 years. The donkey permanent teeth include:

- Three incisors on top and bottom on each side
- One canine on top and bottom on each side (males)
- Three premolars (four if wolf teeth are present) on top and bottom on each side
- Three molars on top and bottom on each side

This grouping results in a total number of approximately 40 teeth in the adult donkey (figs. 6.2 and 6.3). The wolf teeth are the first premolars and have no practical function. They are present in approximately 30% of females and 65% of males.[2] The incisors are used to cut off the plants or food so that it may be taken into the mouth for chewing. The molars and premolars (cheek teeth) chew and grind food between the upper and lower arcades. The incisors and cheek teeth continue to grow throughout the animal's life and are kept in level wear by the opposing tooth above or below. Sharp "points" may develop on the outside edges of the upper cheek teeth and/or inside of the lower cheek teeth. These points can irritate or cut the cheeks or tongue and cause the animal to be reluctant to chew food properly. If a tooth is lost, then

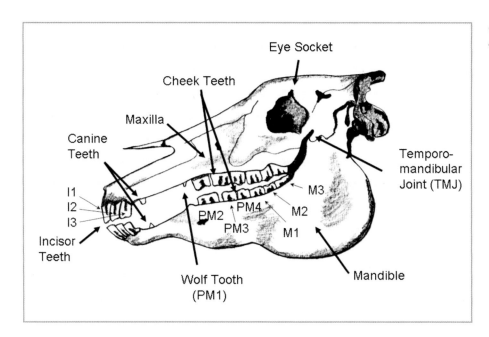

6.2 The normal dentition of the donkey.

the remaining opposite tooth may elongate and interfere with normal chewing motion. Signs of poor tooth conformation include: difficult, prolonged, or slow chewing; dropping food; behavioral issues in the bridle; drooling; quidding (balling up and dropping a wad of food from the mouth due to incomplete chewing) of partially chewed food ; tongue, cheek, or lip injuries; lack of appetite; abnormal mouth odor; weight loss or poor body condition; and colic.

Common tooth problems (in decreasing frequency of occurrence) include: sharp edges on cheek teeth; short, irregular, missing, uneven cheek teeth in old donkeys; loose teeth; and incisor fractures. If the wolf teeth are found in an abnormal position they may angle toward the tongue or become inflamed around the gum, resulting in oral discomfort. Treatment for this is to remove the offending tooth. Overshot jaw conformation may result in uneven wear of the first and last cheek teeth with attendant chewing problems.

An oral exam is best performed by using a speculum to open the mouth. Sedation may be used to facilitate dental procedures and relieve fear and anxiety caused by the equipment or the sensations transmitted to the teeth. As with all procedures on donkeys, patience and a calm attitude are a necessity. Pain medication may be indicated following a prolonged procedure or if mouth sores are discovered. When using a speculum for dental work, it is important not to use it for a prolonged time, particularly in older donkeys as

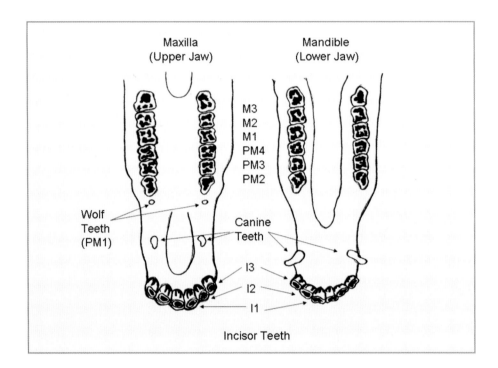

6.3 Occlusal surfaces of the donkey's teeth.

they may have temporomandibular joint (TMJ) problems or cervical spine (neck) arthritis that could be aggravated by forced opening of the mouth. All dental abnormalities may not be correctible at one time; it may be better to do a partial repair and then complete the rest at a later date.

Uneven wear should be identified early and corrected as necessary. Sharp points on cheek teeth may be resolved by a technique known as floating. A long-handled file is introduced into the mouth and rapidly moved in and out as it is angled diagonally to the tooth edges—this blunts and rounds the sharp points. Alternately, power floats may be used if one is very careful not to remove too much tooth.

In older donkeys, loose cheek teeth may be left in place if they are not causing any problem as removal may result in loosening of surrounding teeth. An infected cheek tooth may be pulled with extraction forceps or may require further surgical treatment. Removal of a loose incisor tooth may alleviate discomfort.[3] Dietary management, such as feeding chopped forage products or mashes, can compensate for the inefficiency of loose cheek teeth.

Stomach

When food enters the stomach, contractions of the stomach wall muscles mix it with digestive juices. Hydrochloric acid produced in the stomach continues digestive breakdown of food particles. There is a small amount of microbial fermentation in the esophageal end of the stomach, as well.[4] The capacity of the stomach for food is relatively small, about 8–10 liters for the adult, standard donkey. Food passes out of the stomach 1–2 hours after entry, but the stomach is rarely empty: food remains there for up to three hours after eating has stopped.[5] The stomach's small capacity dictates a need for multiple, small meals or low level, continuous feeding throughout the day to accommodate the most efficient activity of the GI tract. Infrequent feeding or feeding large meals can result in indigestion and colic.

Small Intestine

Partially digested food from the stomach next enters the small intestine, beginning at the duodenum, moving down to the jejunum, and then the ileum. Pancreatic enzymes, intestinal glandular enzymes, and bile from the liver (there is no gall bladder in equines for bile storage) mix here with the food.[6] These enzymes break down proteins, carbohydrates, and fats in the non-fibrous part of the diet throughout the length of the small intestine. Digestive end products such as monosaccharide sugars (glucose, fructose, and galactose), amino acids from protein digestion, and fatty acids from fat digestion are absorbed as peristaltic contractions move the food along. Water, vitamins, and minerals from the intestinal contents are also absorbed into the intestinal circulation.[7]

Large Intestine

Important stages of digestion take place in the large intestine in the cecum and colon. The cecum is a large organ in the donkey as opposed to its human counterpart, the appendix. Micro-organisms, such as bacteria and protozoa, reside within the large intestine to complete the fermentation and digestion of the food. These organisms digest fibrous cellulose, hemicellulose, and lignin products from dietary plant matter. The normal bacterial flora of the hindgut utilize amino acids available from protein digestion; they also synthesize B vitamins and vitamin K needed by the donkey. The food consumed by the donkey determines the species of micro-organisms present in the large intestine, therefore dietary changes result in changing bacterial and protozoal populations.[8] If this happens too rapidly, unstable bacterial populations occur with possible overgrowth of pathogenic organisms; this can lead to diarrhea, laminitis, or colic. It is a good idea to make food changes gradually to avoid such an occurrence. Peristaltic contractions in the large intestine push ingesta (digested food) further along with significant absorption of water, electrolytes (sodium, chloride, potassium, magnesium, calcium, and phosphorus) and nutrients continuing through the hindgut.

Rectum

Waste products from food digestion pass through the rectum in the form of feces. Feces contain a high proportion of microbes along with these undigestible products. Methane gas from microbial fermentation is expelled through the anus. Young animals seed the gut with beneficial microbes by consuming feces (coprophagy). Adults may do so out of boredom.

Hyperlipemia: Liver Disease

Hyperlipemia is defined as an elevation of lipids (fats) in the blood. In addition, this disease is characterized by fatty infiltration of body tissues accompanied by high mortality despite intensive treatment. Early clinical signs are vague and non-specific and easily missed if an owner is not paying close attention to his animals. However, hyperlipemia can be diagnosed quickly and reversed with rapid and early intervention.

Etiology

Hyperlipemia is caused by a negative energy balance in the diet, that is, not enough caloric intake relative to the amount of calories being utilized. A normal calorie source for donkeys is carbohydrates consumed in the form of hay and pasture, and grain if offered. If calories are deficient or if a donkey goes off feed secondary to a disease process, the body relies on using another energy source—it turns to metabolizing fats from adipose (fat) reserves in the body. As stored fat tissue and fatty acids in the bloodstream are metabolized, this process can overwhelm the capacity of the liver's ability to process them, leading to fatty infiltration of liver tissue and subsequent loss of function.

Hyperlipemia has been documented in miniature horses, donkeys, and ponies as a primary disease process and also as a secondary complication to another disease process.[9] Affected donkeys are generally in very good to obese body condition. Some type of physiological or social stress is usually associated with the onset of disease. Examples of inciting stresses include: inclement weather, travel, dietary change, or transfer to a new social situation. Primary diseases associated with secondary hyperlipemia in donkeys and ponies include: dental disease, esophageal obstruction, gastric impaction, intestinal parasitism, and colitis. All these disease situations diminish appetite to limit nutrient supply to the digestive tract.[10] Pregnant or lactating animals are at increased risk for developing hyperlipemia, as are geriatric, female, or obese animals. Alterations in lipid metabolism in obese animals results in an elevated lipid concentration in the blood.

Clinical Signs

In the early stages, the clinical signs of hyperlipemia are often vague. The affected donkey acts lethargic and has a poor appetite, a behavior that is unusual for donkeys; this should alert an owner to investigate a possible cause. If hyperlipemia is a secondary disease entity, primary disease signs may mask it. However, any donkey with a poor appetite should be suspected of having hyperlipemia. The majority of clinical signs observed are a consequence of liver and/or kidney failure. A hyperlipemic donkey may display dullness, lethargy, inappetance, weight loss, edema along the lower abdominal wall, colic, and jaundice. Progression of disease may lead to liver-associated neurologic signs, such as ataxia (incoordination), inability to swallow, head pressing, and circling.

Diagnosis

Hyperlipemia is diagnosed by identifying elevated levels of plasma triglycerides on blood analysis. (See Appendix B for normal donkey blood values, p. 150.) If the condition is severe enough, the plasma may appear milky white when red and white blood cells are allowed to settle out in a blood collection tube. It should be noted that plasma triglycerides elevate normally during gestation, especially in the last trimester. Blood tests that measure liver and kidney function may also be abnormal, supporting the diagnosis. The prognosis of treating donkeys with hyperlipemia is guarded to poor if plasma triglyceride values are in excess of 30 mmol/L.[11]

Treatment

If hyperlipemia is secondary to another disease, then both need to be treated for a successful outcome. The goals of treatment are to correct abnormalities such as dehydration and to reduce plasma lipid levels to normal through nutritional support and minimized stress. A sick donkey should not be separated from its companion if possible. Oral and intravenous nutritional formulations may be administered to correct deficits. Oral medications include water; dextrose, casein, or dehydrated cottage cheese; pelleted or cubed feeds; and electrolytes and vitamins.

Affected donkeys should be encouraged to eat by offering highly palatable feeds and hand feeding if necessary. It is critical to get calories into these animals to try to restore their metabolism. Other drugs used by your veterinarian to treat this condition might include injectable anabolic steroids, multivitamins, and insulin. Use of corticosteroid drugs is contraindicated as they will exacerbate the hyperlipemia.

Prevention

Basic, sound nutritional management is key to avoiding this potentially fatal disease. Donkeys should be provided adequate calories in the form of carbohydrates; however, obesity should always be avoided. Stressful situations should be minimized and in particular pay close attention to at-risk donkeys, such as female, obese, and/or pregnant individuals. Nutritional support must be provided to sick animals suffering from situations like colic or esophageal obstruction.

Colic

Colic is defined simply as "abdominal pain." It is not a specific disease entity as potential sources of colic are many. Common gastrointestinal sources for colic include: the distal esophagus (esophageal choke); the stomach (impaction or ulcers); the small intestine (blockage, inflammation, or torsion); the large intestine (impaction, displacement or torsion, or colitis or ulcerative colitis); and the liver (swelling from infection or tumors). Other sources of pain in the abdomen can arise from the kidney (swelling with infection, tumors, or stones), the ovaries in jennets (possibly from tumors), or at the time of foaling.

Clinical Signs

In general, donkeys are very stoic especially when compared to most horses. With this in mind, any evidence of signs of abdominal pain should be considered significant. A donkey that will not eat is a sick donkey and the cause of the lack of appetite should be investigated. Any abnormal behavior should be cause for concern. Knowing the normal behavior of each individual donkey helps you identify when something is wrong.

Clinical signs associated with colic are related to abdominal discomfort. Often an affected donkey stretches out as if he wants to urinate or defecate, leading to an often incorrect assumption that the donkey is unable to urinate or may be constipated. Other clinical signs of pain include pawing with the front feet; turning to look at the flank; lying down (this may be confused with sleeping in tired animals); getting up and down frequently; falling down (may be falsely diagnosed as an inability to stand due to neurologic disease); rolling; sweating; quivering; and flehmen (rolling up) of the upper lip. Lack of appetite, backing up to a wall or paddock fence, kicking at the abdomen, groaning, or assuming a dog-sitting position are other behaviors seen with colic. Halitosis (bad smelling breath) often accompanies ileus (lack of gut motility) in donkeys.[12]

Cardiovascular signs associated with colic include elevated heart rate (normal range is 35–60 beats per minute) and respiratory rate (normal averages 20 breaths per minute). Dehydration is also present in severe cases and may be tested by pinching the skin over the eye socket between the index finger and thumb. In normally hydrated animals, the pinched skin returns to flat within two seconds. Abnormal oral mucous membrane color may also be seen in severe cases with the normal pink color replaced by pale pink or dark red. Abnormal circulation is also evidenced by capillary refill time greater than three seconds when gums are blanched with finger pressure.

Gastrointestinal Tract Abnormalities

Most colic originates from abnormalities of the GI tract. Normally, the GI tract is in a constant state of motion as the digestive processes progress. The equine GI tract reacts to abnormal digestion or lack of movement when something causes irritation or interferes with normal peristalsis to slow its movement. This may result in distention of the intestine as digesta, fluid, or gas builds up. Obstructions cause bowel size to increase upstream of the blockage. The bowel wall and mesentery (tissue support for small intestines) stretch as a result and this compresses veins in the intestinal wall and leads to pain. Locally, capillary pressure and filtration rate increase to cause edema of the bowel wall along with increased secretion of fluid into the intestine. Pressure increases are accompanied by pain and decreased bowel motility, with an unending cycle if timely veterinary intervention does not occur The goals of standard treatments for colic are to relieve the increased pressure, relieve pain, and return peristaltic contractions to normal.

Types of GI Tract Colic

There are a few main types of colic associated with the GI tract. Gas colic results from a buildup of gas usually from stress or a dietary change. Gas colic usually responds readily to pain medications and passage of a nasogastric tube from the nose into the stomach to relieve pressure.

Impaction colic occurs when feed material within the GI tract forms into a blockage. This is usually associated with inadequate water intake, poor quality feed, dehydration from climatic conditions, deficient water availability, or secondary to a disease process. Intestinal impactions often involve the large colon and the small colon. One study in the United Kingdom found fibrous balls of poorly chewed, entangled forage up to 8 by 15 cm in dimension that were lodged inside the bowel. This obstruction led to progressive ileus (lack of motility) and endotoxemia (effects from toxins that enter the circulation from dying intestinal bacteria).[13] If diagnosed early, impaction colic may respond to conservative medical treatment in the field but some cases also require intensive intravenous fluid therapy and potential surgery.

An obstruction may develop that prevents ingesta from moving down the intestinal tract. This may occur due to: displacement of the small or large bowel from its normal position; tumors, such as fatty masses (lipomas) in older donkeys; twists of the bowel along the longitudinal or vertical axis (accompanied by severe pain); a diaphragmatic hernia (intestine passes through the diaphragm to become trapped in the thoracic cavity); or any bowel entrapment in an abnormal location. Simple indigestion from abnormal food intake may progress to an obstruction if intestinal peristalsis is slowed. It is common to see donkeys roll with no untoward effects but at a time when circulation and intestinal peristalsis might be compromised, it is possible for the bowel to displace into an abnormal position or twist upon its axis; this may occur even in a standing animal.

Esophageal choke is an obstructive digestive tract problem, occurring in the esophagus, not in the respiratory tract. Typically, improper or inadequate chewing from dental problems or greedy behavior that causes a donkey to bolt its feed are reasons why the initial steps of chewing might be bypassed; incomplete chewing has the potential for feed to jam in the esophagus. In other cases, rapidly consumed pelleted feed may swell when mixed with small amounts of saliva on its way down the esophagus. The site of obstruction is variable, but the donkey will display any number of signs: drooling, stretching out its neck, pawing, flehmen, saliva mixed with feed draining from the nostrils, or coughing and gagging. Some individuals display typical colic signs due to choke. If a case of esophageal choke does not resolve spontaneously within an hour, then it is necessary for your veterinarian to treat the donkey to try to push the lodged mass into the stomach by passage of a nasogastric tube. This is done with care so as not to damage the esophagus. On occasion, the mass may defy these efforts, and warm water and a small amount of detergent may be carefully used to soften the mass. Anti-inflammatory drugs such as flunixin meglumine are often administered for the associated pain and swelling.

Severity of Clinical Signs

Increased severity of signs is usually associated with increased severity of the problem. Donkeys are usually stoic, but the pain tolerance of individual animals varies. Severe pain signs may be associated with a simple problem, and mild signs may be associated with a severe problem. In general, donkeys may usually require up to 25% more pain medication than a horse of equal size.

First Aid Treatment

It is okay for a donkey to lie down with colic but it is not okay for him to roll. A twisted bowel can occur in a standing donkey, but rolling has more potential to change a mild problem into a severe one by causing large excursions of the compromised bowel through the abdomen. Walking a colicking donkey for a short time (20–30 minutes) serves to distract the animal from the pain but this should not be the only treatment used for colic and it should not be overdone. Oral antacids such as Pepto-Bismol,™ Mylanta®, and Milk of Magnesia may be administered in simple cases under the advisement of your veterinarian. A turkey baster can be used to administer 60–120 cc (one to two turkey basters full) per adult donkey.

Nonsteroidal anti-inflammatory drugs (NSAIDS) are used for pain relief for colic. Injectable flunixin meglumine can provide rapid pain relief for a simple colic when given intravenously. Although labeled for intramuscular use, the injectable form has occasionally caused serious and potentially life-threatening infections with *Clostridial* bacteria when given in the muscle to horses. Oral flunixin meglumine or phenylbutazone products have hours of lag time to be absorbed from the bowel and this takes even longer when bowel motility and circulation is compromised as with colic.

The best advice is for an owner to call the vet early when any colic signs are recognized. The vet can usually correct simple medical problems if managed early before progressing to a surgical condition. However, some colic cases are in immediate need of surgery regardless of rapidity of medical intervention. Survival rate for surgical treatment of colic is directly related to the severity of clinical signs at the onset, and how soon corrective action is undertaken.

Standard Vet Exams

The standard parameters checked in colicking donkeys are: heart and respiratory rate, rectal temperature, capillary refill time, hydration status, and stethoscope examination for GI tract sounds. The veterinarian will also percuss (ping with a finger over the area listened to with the stethoscope) the abdomen to detect the presence of gas. Expect the vet to pass a nasogastric tube to check for gas and fluid distention of the stomach and to provide relief if present. Fluid reflux from the stomach is abnormal and its presence indicates a likely obstruction somewhere in the upper GI tract from either a mechanical blockage or a physiological blockage related to pain that has slowed intestinal contractions.

A rectal exam to assess the status of the reachable bowel may be performed if the case appears to be complicated or is not improving after treatment. This diagnostic procedure carries a risk of bowel perforation of the animal or injury to the veterinarian or animal handler; it is often not possible to perform a rectal exam in small donkeys, especially for a person with large hands and arms. The information a rectal exam provides is valuable. It is used to assess presence and character of the manure and to evaluate for distension of bowel components. It may reveal an impaction and is useful to assess intra-abdominal pressure increase that accompanies large bowel distention. Manure may be tested for sand at the farm by mixing a few fecal balls with water in a plastic glove or baggie to check for settling of sand. Manure may also be saved for a fecal exam. Ultrasound equipment may be used to assess distention of bowel segments not able to be palpated per rectum.

Differentiating Surgical from Medical Colic

One of the most important jobs of the veterinarian during examination of a colic case is to assess whether the animal needs surgery to correct the condition causing the colic. The majority (95%) of colic cases are treated successfully with simple medical treatment if diagnosed early. Indications for surgical intervention in a colic case include: presence of pain that is uncontrollable with analgesics, progressive distension of the abdomen, deteriorating cardiovascular status, or discovering abnormal results on an abdominal tap. An abdominal tap may be performed in the field or at a referral facility after the donkey has been sent for advanced treatment. Early referral of surgical cases greatly increases the survival rate.

Simple Field Medical Treatments

Simple medical treatments that are useful in alleviating the signs of colic include: IV flunixin meglumine for pain relief, passage of a nasogastric tube to decompress the stomach, and administration of fluids and laxative medications by stomach tube based on physical exam findings. Warm water is used to correct dehydration and stimulate gut motility. Mineral oil is sometimes administered through the tube to serve as a lubricant for intestinal contents and to absorb toxic products of abnormal digestion. Other valuable laxative treatments that might be administered through a stomach tube include magnesium (Epsom) salts, psyllium, and/or veterinary surfactant used to break down gas and help to soften a suspected impaction. Electrolytes may be added to tubed fluids or drinking water as they are important for normal gut motility.

Most donkeys respond to simple medical treatments. If not, it is likely that the problem requires advanced medical treatment or surgery. If the donkey continues to be in pain, depressed, or is not showing clinical improvement or passing manure, consideration should be given to transporting the donkey to a referral hospital in a timely fashion. If the donkey gets worse after being given oral medications, suspect some type of obstruction, which most likely will require surgery to correct. Impactions usually respond well at first, but require retreatment later in the day or on the next day. An impaction may respond eventually to intravenous fluid therapy without surgical intervention.

Treatments at Referral Hospitals

The owner should expect referral hospital veterinarians to repeat the basic examination procedures to compare the donkey's clinical signs with those discovered before referral. Advanced procedures include: diagnostic ultrasound exam of the abdomen; an abdominal tap and fluid analysis to check for infection or bowel wall compromise; and blood analysis of PCV, protein, and electrolytes to help select appropriate fluids for IV therapy. Performance of an abdominal tap (abdominocentesis) in donkeys is often complicated by retroperitoneal fat that can be up to 15 cm thick on the midline of the ventral abdomen where the tap is done.[14] Medical or surgical treatment will be selected based on the results of these procedures and as elected by the owner.

Sometimes a donkey improves during the trailer ride to the hospital. It is important to transport the animal early to improve chances of obtaining the best outcome if advanced medical or surgical treatment is an option. At the referral hospital, the owner may elect to pursue medical treatment only, or authorize humane euthanasia if medical treatment is not successful or the outlook is guarded to poor. Another option is for the donkey to have abdominal exploratory surgery for identification of the cause of the colic; then the surgeon can proceed with correction or euthanize the animal on the operating table if the prognosis is hopeless. Statistics associated with surgical treatment of colic in horses reveal an overall, initial survival rate approximating 75%, meaning that 25% of cases fail. The recurrence rate of colic varies relative to the severity of problem and the extent of surgery required to correct the problem. Post-operative formation of adhesions (scar tissue) between abdominal organs and loops of bowel may predispose animals to future colic attacks.

Factors Associated with Increased Risk of Colic in Horses

Predisposing factors for colic have not been published for donkeys. It is worthwhile to discuss predisposing factors in horses as they might also be applicable. Increasing age increases the incidence of colic. In horses, there are known predispositions to colic conditions. Intussusception (a piece of bowel telescopes into another adjacent piece) is associated with younger horses or with tapeworm infection. Inflammation and scarring by larval migration may elicit colic in horses less than 6 years old.[15] Strangulating lipomas occur in older horses. Mares are subject to uterine torsion and colon torsion in the initial days following foaling. Stallions and recently gelded horses are susceptible to herniation of intestinal contents through the scrotum. Young, miniature horses may be subject to fecaliths (mass of feces surrounding a nidus or nucleus of foreign material) and small colon impactions.

Medical history relevant to colic attacks includes incidence of previous colic attacks, especially if previous abdominal surgery was performed. Farm management factors may increase chances of colic including: recent change of diet, feeding "excessive" amounts of grain, poor quality or restricted access to water, high stocking density, drastic changes in activity level, poor dental care (choke and large colon impaction), and inadequate parasite control practices. Weather changes, such as cold to hot and vice versa may predispose some animals to colic. This may be a result of dehydration and sweating, inadequate water consumption, or changes in barometric pressure associated with storms.

Two studies at the Donkey Sanctuary in England have shed more light on the role of gastrointestinal impactions in donkey colic. Cox et al reported that 54.8% of suspect or confirmed cases of colic were caused by GI impactions, with 39.8% being at the pelvic flexure, where the large colon folds back on itself on the left side of the abdomen.[16] Factors associated with increased risk included: older donkeys, those fed extra rations, previous history of colic, light body weight, musculoskeletal problems, and dental disease. The study also confirmed a seasonal pattern with autumn peaks and troughs in spring and early summer possibly associated with changes in husbandry.[17]

Summary

- The anatomy of the donkey's digestive system is similar to that of the horse. The major components work in unison to make donkeys very efficient converters of consumed forage even if it is low in digestible quality or nutritional composition. Digestive tract components include the mouth, esophagus, stomach, small intestine, large intestine (cecum and colon), and the rectum.

- Common tooth problems in donkeys (in decreasing frequency of occurrence) include: sharp edges on cheek teeth; short, irregular, missing, uneven cheek teeth in old donkeys; loose teeth; and incisor fractures.

- The stomach's small capacity dictates a need for multiple small meals or low level, continuous feeding throughout the day to accommodate the most efficient activity of the gastrointestinal (GI) tract. Infrequent feeding or feeding large meals can result in indigestion and colic.

- Partially digested food from the stomach enters the small intestine, beginning at the duodenum, moving down to the jejunum, and then to the ileum. Pancreatic enzymes, intestinal glandular enzymes, and bile from the liver (there is no gall bladder in equines for bile storage) mix here with the food.

- Important stages of digestion take place in the large intestine in the cecum and colon. Waste products from food digestion pass through the rectum in the form of feces. Feces contain a high proportion of microbes along with these undigestible products.

- Hyperlipemia is defined as an elevation of lipids (fats) in the blood. This disease is characterized by fatty infiltration of body tissues accompanied by high mortality despite intensive treatment. Early clinical signs are vague and non-specific and easily missed if an owner is not paying close attention to his animals. It can be diagnosed quickly and reversed with rapid and early intervention. Basic, sound nutritional management is the key to avoiding this potentially fatal disease.

- Colic is defined simply as "abdominal pain." It is not a specific disease entity as potential sources of colic are many. Common gastrointestinal sources for colic include: the distal esophagus (esophageal choke); the stomach (impaction or ulcers); the small intestine (blockage, inflammation, or torsion); the large intestine (impaction, displacement or torsion, or colitis or ulcerative colitis); and the liver (swelling from infection or tumors).

- Other sources of pain in the abdomen can arise from the kidney (swelling with infection, tumors, or stones); the ovaries in jennets (possibly from tumors); or at the time of foaling.

- Clinical signs associated with colic are related to abdominal discomfort. These may include: stretching as if to urinate or defecate; pawing with the front feet; turning to look at the flank; lying down; getting up and down frequently; falling down; rolling; sweating; quivering; flehmen (rolling up) of the upper lip; lack of appetite; backing up to a wall or paddock fence; kicking at the abdomen; groaning; or assuming a dog-sitting position.

- Cardiovascular signs associated with colic include elevated heart rate and respiratory rate. Dehydration, abnormal mucous membrane color, and prolonged capillary refill time may be present in severe cases.

- The goals of standard treatments for colic are to relieve the increased pressure, relieve pain, and return peristaltic contractions to normal.

- The standard parameters checked in colicking donkeys are: heart and respiratory rate; rectal temperature; capillary refill time; hydration status; and stethoscope examination for GI tract sounds.

- One of the most important jobs of the veterinarian during examination of a colic case is to assess whether the animal needs surgery to correct the condition causing the colic. The majority (95%) of colic cases are treated successfully with simple medical treatment if diagnosed early.

- Predisposing factors for colic have not been published for donkeys. Predisposing factors in horses might also be applicable to donkeys.

References

1. Thiemann, AK. "Dentistry in the Elderly Donkey." Donkey Clinical Welfare in Practice Meeting Proceedings. October 2007, The Donkey Sanctuary, UK.

2. See note 1 above.

3. See note 1 above.

4. Pearson, RA. "Nutrition and Feeding of Donkeys in Veterinary Care of Donkeys." Matthews, NS, and Taylor, TS. International Veterinary Information Service, Ithaca, NY (www.ivis.org).

5. See note 1 above.

6. See note 4 above.

7. See note 4 above.

8. See note 4 above.

9. Boyce, M. "Hyperlipemia in Miniature Horses." *Stanislaus Journal of Biochemical Reviews*, May 1999.

10. Watson, TDG. "The Hyperlipemic Donkey: Recognition, Treatment and Advances in Management." http://www.manc.umd.edu/2006_Complete_Proceedings.pdf

11. See note 10 above.

12. Mair, T; Divers, T; Ducharme, N, WB. *Manual of Equine Gastroenterology.* Saunders, New York, 2002.

13. Crane, M. "Colic and Geriatric Disease." Donkey Welfare in Clinical Practice Meeting Proceedings, UK, 2007.

14. See note 12 above.

15. See note 9 above.

16. See note 13 above.

17. Cox, R, et al. "Epidemiology of impaction colic in donkeys in the UK." *BMC Veterinary Research.* 2007, 3:1-11.

Musculoskeletal System

The donkey and its joints are subjected to daily wear and tear during work, exercise, and even when grazing or standing still. The joints of the musculoskeletal system absorb shock, permit relatively frictionless movement, and bear the weight of a body that may weigh up to 1,200–1,500 lbs (550–650 kg).

Joint Classifications

There are three types of joints in the body: fibrous, cartilaginous, and synovial.

Fibrous joints are least likely to be afflicted with disease because they are more or less immobile. They include the joints in the skull and those between the shafts of some long bones, as for example, the connection between the splint bones and the cannon bones.

Cartilaginous joints don't have a high propensity for disease due to limited movement. One example of this type is located at the growth plates of the long bones of the limbs where specialized cartilage there converts to bone to extend leg length during the donkey's growing years. Another example lies between the pelvis and the sacral vertebrae at the sacroiliac joint.

Synovial joints (fig. 7.1) are the most likely to suffer disease and injury because they are the most active. They consist of two bone ends covered by articular (joint) cartilage, which is smooth and resilient and when properly lubricated, enables frictionless movement of the joint. Injury of the soft tissue associated with a synovial joint may result in more watery and dilute joint fluid; the resulting increased friction results in more wear on the cartilage and synovial membrane (joint lining). Stability of high-motion synovial joints is maintained by a fibrous joint capsule, which is attached to and connects the two long bones that form the joint, and also by collateral ligaments located on either side of most joints—these are important soft tissue components

7.1 A typical synovial joint.

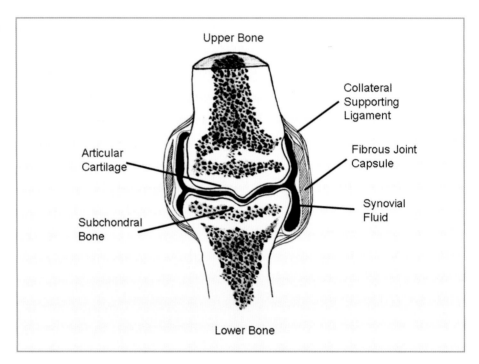

in the fetlock, knee, elbow, hock, and stifle joints. Some joints have internal ligaments within them (e.g., cruciate ligaments in the stifle) to help mechanically stabilize the joint.

The lubrication of synovial joints protects them against friction, which causes joint wear and damage. The joint capsule contains an inner lining called the synovial membrane that secretes the synovial fluid that lubricates the joint. Hyaluronic acid (sodium hyaluronate or hyaluronan) in the fluid lubricates the synovial membrane. In some cases of joint disease, there is a depletion of lubricating joint fluid subsequent to inflammation of the joint from injury or use over time. Increased friction within the joint amplifies wear of the cartilage and contributes to advancement of osteoarthritis (degenerative joint disease). The forelimbs bear 60–65% of a donkey's weight and are thus subjected to greater concussive effects than the rear legs, especially when a donkey is moving at speed. Depending on the type of work a donkey is asked to perform, the stress load may shift more to the rear limbs. Poor limb and body conformation place undue stress on joint structures even at the walk, and this stress is greatly magnified with poor conformation, speed, hard work, athletic maneuvers, or jumping.

Each joint is stabilized by a complex network of tendons, ligaments, and muscles. When all is well, this complex network enables a joint to function in a smooth, synchronized fashion. When any part of the network malfunctions because of injury or disease, medical or surgical treatment might be necessary.

Forelimb Joints

Because the lower leg joints of the front limbs receive most of the concussive stress during movement, they are most prone to injury and disease. By the time concussion reaches the elbow and shoulder, its effects have been dissipated effectively by the other joints. Shoulder and elbow joints are less prone to concussive injury and disease.

Hind Limb Joints

Lower leg joints of the hind limbs are similar to those in the front limb. The hock or tarsus is actually composed of four separate joints, with only the top one providing significant motion. These multiple joints are held together by a complex set of ligaments. The stifle joint (analogous to the human knee) is the donkey's largest synovial joint and is composed of three separate joint compartments. The hip joint has a ball-and-socket construction stabilized by strong bands of ligaments. The upper end of the femur fits into a socket on the pelvic bone.

Joint Disease

Donkeys have joint problems because we often ask them to do things they were not designed to do. Concussive force is concentrated on joints of the front legs when, for example, a donkey jumps an obstacle and lands on his front feet.

Traumatic arthritis is a diverse collection of pathological and clinical states that develop after single or repetitive episodes of trauma. Components of traumatic arthritis may include: synovitis (inflammation of the joint lining); capsulitis (inflammation of the fibrous joint capsule); strain or sprain (injury to the supporting ligaments of the joint); and fractures of bones within the joint. Trauma creates physical and biochemical damage to the articular cartilage. In some donkeys,

Suggested Reading

• Stashak T. Adams *Lameness in Horses*. 5th ed. Lippincott, 2001.

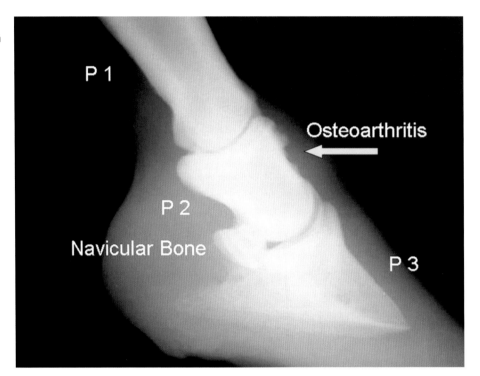

7.2 A radiograph showing calcification associated with chronic, severe arthritis.

joint injury and disease occur after years of stress (fig. 7.2). These would be the donkeys with correct conformation whose joints were strong and supple enough to withstand trauma for a long time before weakening. In others, joint injury and disease might occur after only a single traumatic incident. These might be the donkeys with conformation anomalies that predispose them to problems. It is important to pay attention to conformation and the effects of repetitive or inappropriate exercise.

Available treatments for joint inflammation are few and may be employed as a combination of options. Rest is the most simple and often overlooked treatment. It is simply a change in the exercise level or use of the animal and should be part of any treatment plan. Anti-inflammatory medications, such as flunixin meglumine and phenylbutazone, are used to decrease inflammation in joint structures. Intra-articular (within the joint) corticosteroids are used to decrease inflammation of the soft tissue structures of a synovial joint. Joint-specific drugs, such as intramuscular or intra-articular polysulfated glycosaminoglycans (Adequan® by Luitpold) or intravenous or intra-articular hyaluronic acid (Legend® by Bayer) or intra-articular injection of one of many other available hyaluronic acid products , may be used to decrease joint inflammation and aid in return to function of soft tissue and cartilage structures. Usually, a combination of these is used to treat arthritis, but always include rest and consider a job change for a donkey with a chronic condition.

Lameness Diagnosis

Lameness is defined as an abnormality of gait caused by pain and/or restriction of movement. Lameness is graded on the following scale:

- Grade 1 = mild, inconsistent lameness when trotted in a straight line
- Grade 2 = obvious, consistent, mild lameness with pelvic hike or head nod
- Grade 3 = pronounced pelvic hike with a head nod
- Grade 4 = moderate lameness with an extreme head nod and pelvic hike; donkey will still trot
- Grade 5 = non-weight bearing (do not trot if non weight-bearing while standing)

Most causes of lameness fall into the following categories:

- Degenerative: e.g. degenerative joint disease (DJD, or osteoarthritis)
- Developmental: e.g. osteochondrosis (OCD), physitis (also called epiphysitis)
- Metabolic: e.g. laminitis (founder), exertional rhabdomyolysis (tying up)
- Mechanical overload of a structure: sudden, massive overload or repetitive, marginal overload (wear and tear)
- Infectious: e.g. foot abscess, infected wounds, cellulitis, joint infection
- Inflammatory: most of the specific causes of lameness have an inflammatory component
- Traumatic: injury (external trauma)

Visual Observation

Visual observation is the key to identifying which leg is lame. An abnormal stance, such as pointing the toe, resting one leg more than another, or a positional change of the fetlock may give clues as to which leg is affected. It is also possible that more than one leg is affected and the animal may walk or trot stiffly all over. Other signs of lameness include abnormal movement (head nod) for forelimb lameness or a hip hike for a hind limb lameness. A reduced arc of foot flight associated with lameness is often seen as stiffness or reluctance to flex the limb normally. There may also be a shortened stride length or shortened swing phase (forward motion of the limb) of the stride. Abnormal foot placement may also be observed, as for example, landing toe first to reduce pressure on the heel.

Evaluation of Gait

In the course of diagnosing lameness, the gait should be evaluated on a level, even surface at the walk and also at the trot for evidence of asymmetry or abnormalities. The donkey should also be observed while moving in a straight line and on a circle (led, longed, or in a round pen). During this exam the donkey should be on a loose lead or longe line so that the head motion is unrestricted. It is important to watch the donkey in both directions on the circle, from the side, from the front, and from the rear on both hard and soft surfaces as lameness may be more obvious with one of these circumstances. Adding the weight of a rider, if appropriate, often exacerbates most lameness.

Investigating the Cause of a Lameness

Locating the specific area involved requires two basic tools: the eyes and the hands. The skills of observation, palpation, and manipulation are employed during the exam. Observation includes looking for symmetry between left and right legs or between the inside and outside of a normally symmetrical structure.

When asymmetry is found, it should be determined whether it is due to enlargement (swelling) or reduction in tissue mass. Palpation involves feeling for heat, swelling, pain, and changes in tone or texture of the tissue. Swellings should be characterized as hard, firm, soft, or fluid-filled. Manipulation involves moving the structure or tissue through its normal range of motion to check for pain, altered range of motion (increase or decrease), and crepitus (a grating, grinding, or crackling sensation). The examiner should use these tools to identify the five basic signs of inflammation: pain, heat, swelling, redness, and loss of function.

The foot is the most common site of lameness. One should examine the hoof wall for symmetry and integrity (cracks, bulges), and should check the sole for defects or foreign objects, as well as examining for discharge, discoloration, or odor. Carefully examine the shoe and nails for abnormalities. The coronary band should be checked for pain, swellings, or indentations. Check the heel bulbs and sole for response to thumb pressure. Manipulation is used to try to move the heels independently. Digital pulses (at the lower fetlock or pastern) should be palpated for increases indicative of inflammation in the lower limb that they supply. The examiner should tap the hoof wall with a small hammer or tool to check for a pain response. Hoof testers applied across the heels, sole, and frog check for signs of pain; discomfort is communicated by the donkey by tensing limb or neck muscles or by withdrawal of the affected limb.

The joints are another common source of lameness. Observation of swelling and position (angulation) is used in the diagnostic procedure. Finger palpation of joints may reveal the nature of the swelling, heat, pain, and/or enlarged joint pouches. Manipulation of joints includes flexion (bending) and extension (straightening), and checking for pain and altered range of motion to aid in localizing the source of a problem.

When examining bones, tendons, and ligaments, use the tools of observation for swelling, palpation for heat and pain, and manipulation for evidence of pain, instability, or crepitus. Muscles are examined in a similar fashion. Muscle atrophy (wasting) indicates a loss of function for at least a couple of weeks. Forelimb muscle atrophy is often most evident in the scapular muscles, while hind limb atrophy is most evident in the croup region in the gluteal muscles. Loss of function in one leg and its relative disuse due to lameness may result in asymmetry in the muscle mass as compared to the same muscles on the uninvolved limb. The neck and back consist of a complex series of bones, joints, tendons, ligaments, and muscles, which may be painful on palpation or manipulation.

Ill-fitting tack, especially the saddle, can cause soreness in the back muscles and over the withers, possibly resulting in lameness. Poorly seated or unbalanced riders and related mouth injuries due to tack, poor equitation skills, or from dental disease abnormalities may be interpreted as lameness. Other possible sources of lameness include the skin—in the case of infections or punctures—and the nervous system components of brain, spinal cord, or peripheral nerves.

Interpreting Examination Findings

The pain response found on manipulation or palpation must be repeatable to be valid. Repeat evaluation of a suspect area should reveal the same (or greater) response to palpation or manipulation each time. The pain response may be subtle (tensing up, turning the head to look, moving away from the hand), but if it is repeatable, it is probably significant. Assuming the opposite leg is normal, use it for comparison to help interpret the significance of the exam findings. Some animals may become desensitized with repeated attempts to elicit pain in a suspect area. This ends up with the donkey failing to exhibit any response although an actual area of injury is being squeezed and probed.

Most lameness problems involve a structure at the level of or below the knee or hock. The foot is the source of many lameness conditions. Once a source of lameness is identified do not overlook other structures or additional injuries that may also be involved in the lameness. A specific diagnosis often is not possible without a thorough veterinary examination, diagnostic nerve blocks, and diagnostic imaging.

A veterinarian will conduct a full physical examination. Joint flexion tests are also performed to stress joints and associated structures in an effort to exacerbate the signs of observed lameness. Lower leg flexion tests stress the fetlock and below. Upper leg flexion tests in front stress the carpus and elbow and, in the rear, the hock, stifle, and hip. Hock arthritis often starts in the lower inside joints and direct pressure over this area may evoke a withdrawal reaction to help localize a problem.

The veterinarian may use regional anesthetic nerve blocks to selectively numb areas of the lower limbs to localize the source of lameness. These findings may be accompanied by a radiographic examination of the suspect area of concern. Individual joint blocks may be used to rule problems in or out within the joint; this is an invasive procedure involving direct injection of local anesthetic into the joint with attendant risks of bacterial infection. One should avoid needle punctures into joints because of the damage done by the puncture and also the risk of introducing bacteria into the joint, which may result in an infection. If this technique is deemed appropriate it should be carried out by an experienced veterinarian under aseptic conditions.

Many musculoskeletal injuries respond well to rest and anti-inflammatory medications, but in a refractory case that does not respond, there is a selection of imaging modalities available to investigate the problem. Diagnostic imaging is useful to evaluate conditions such as arthritis, possible fractures, and laminitis. Radiography (using X-ray generating equipment) is used to evaluate bones and joints. Ultrasonography is used for diagnosis of soft-tissue problems, such as tendon and ligament injuries, and joint surface damage. Thermography is a technique that images and maps out surface temperatures of the body to identify areas of inflammation (increased temperature) or reduced blood flow (decreased temperature). Nuclear scintigraphy is useful for identifying soft tissue inflammation and bone or joint problems. This entails injection of a radioactive substance into the bloodstream where it is distributed throughout the body, typically collecting in areas of increased circulation or bone remodeling. The radioactive marker is identified using a special gamma camera, which records the radioactive emissions where the marker collects. Computerized tomography (CT scanning) is useful for examination of any tissue, but is mostly used for bone problems. Magnetic resonance imaging (MRI) is used mostly for soft tissue and joint surface examinations. These latter two modalities provide precise information, but they are also very expensive and can only image limb areas from the hock or knee down. General anesthesia is usually necessary to maintain absolute stillness of the donkey as it is positioned within human MRI machines for the exam.

Laminitis

Laminitis is an inflammatory disease of the laminar tissue, which connects the coffin bone to the inside of the hoof wall. In donkeys, it is often related to a digestive change with the resulting damage due to circulatory insufficiency to the lamina. Founder may be used synonymously for laminitis but the word is nautical in origin referring to the sinking of the coffin bone inside the hoof capsule after the laminae have been weakened and tear. Most cases of laminitis are not associated with this sinking phenomenon.

Causes

Laminitis is a secondary disease, most often occurring after a digestive disturbance, such as grain overload, rich pasture consumption, or severe diarrhea as seen with bacterial colitis caused by *Salmonella* or a viral agent. A common scenario for the development of laminitis is the overweight donkey turned out on lush grass. Other inciting causes include toxemia, such as that following untreated, retained fetal membranes (placenta) post-foaling and the resulting endometritis (uterine infection). Drugs like corticosteroids (for example, dexamethasone) or diseases like Cushing's disease or associated hypothyroidism (underproduction of thyroid hormone) have been associated with laminitis in horses and may also affect donkeys. Mechanical laminitis may be the result of "road founder" from excess concussion related to exercise, whether it be on a hard road or overuse on any surface.

Clinical Signs of Acute Laminitis

The stoic nature of donkeys might allow laminitis to advance long before showing evidence of foot pain. Most cases are chronic with clinical signs only evident during an acute flare up. Foot pain may be manifested as the donkey being reluctant to move even when asked, as if he is "glued to the ground." Other rule outs for this behavior include colic (see p. 76) or tying-up syndrome. An affected donkey may stand with the weight shifted to the rear legs and the front limbs positioned forward of normal. This stance may also be seen with a painful front foot abscess or sore heels, although in those cases, generally only one foot is involved. A laminitic donkey may spend a lot of time lying down as in colic or what might be seen with a neurologic problem. Or,

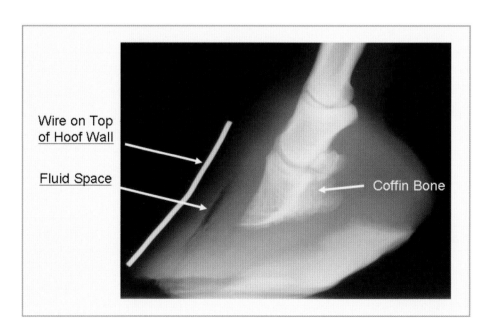

7.3 Lateral radiograph of the coffin bone. The dorsal (front) surface of the coffin bone (P3) is parallel to the top portion of the hoof wall, but the bottom portion of the hoof wall is deviating upward from imbalanced growth due to decreased circulation in the toe. A space of fluid density is visible where the hoof wall laminae have been severely damaged.

Wire on Top of Hoof Wall

Fluid Space

Coffin Bone

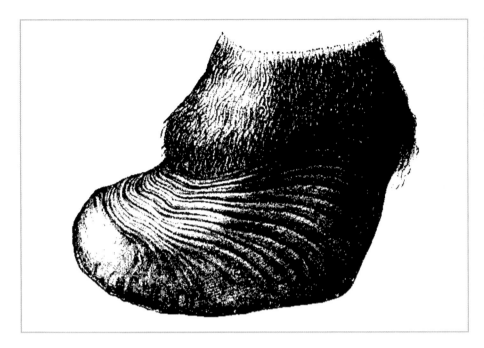

7.4 Lateral view of the foot of a donkey with chronic laminitis. Note the diverging hoof wall growth rings from slowed growth at the front of the hoof while the rear of the hoof continues at the normal rate.

the donkey may exhibit a stiff gait at the walk, preferring to load the heels, as if "walking on eggs." This typical gait also develops in a donkey that is foot-sore due to a recent and over-zealous hoof trim or if bruised by traversing uneven or rocky ground.

Increased digital pulses are a common component of laminitis and may also occur with a foot abscess, severe bruise, or lower leg injury. The greater the laminar swelling that is present, the stronger the digital pulses. Increased hoof temperature may be appreciated, most often in both front feet. With careful examination of the bottom of the foot, bruising may be detected at the white line (junction of the hoof wall and the sole). Pain may be evident by sensitivity to hoof testers over the sole at and around the apex (point) of the frog. Early on in the episode, some donkeys may not show sensitivity to hoof testers. If damage is worse in one foot, then lameness may only be evident in that foot.

Significant laminar damage results in separation of the hoof wall from the coffin bone (P3) and fluid and/or bleeding beneath the hoof wall (fig. 7.3). The coffin bone may rotate or sink; the degree of damage is best determined by radiographs. Positional changes (rotation or sinking) of the coffin bone within the hoof capsule result in further circulatory compromise to the foot and without intervention, damage to the laminae may continue.

Clinical Signs of Chronic Laminitis

Clinical signs of laminitis may include: misshapen hooves with diverging rings (fig. 7.4); a very stiff, short strided gait; periodic or recurrent lameness, especially in the front feet; deviation between the coffin bones and dorsal hoof wall on radiographs; demineralization and deformity of the coffin bone; and evidence of a dropped sole. When looking at the foot, there may be an area of vertical hoof growth below the coronary band, indicative of the position of the top surface of the coffin bone inside the hoof.

Treatment

The basis for treatment is to support the coffin bone (P3 or third phalanx) to prevent rotation and sinking. First aid treatment for laminitis may include pulling shoes if present along with temporary frog support (Lily Pads®, or roll gauze, or a thick piece of blue or pink Styrofoam board cut to the size of the bottom of the foot and taped in place.)

Corrective trimming to reestablish the normal position of the coffin bone within the hoof is carried out as determined by radiographs of the feet (fig. 7.5). I discuss this further on p. 99.

7.5 A radiograph showing significant downward rotation of the coffin bone (P3).

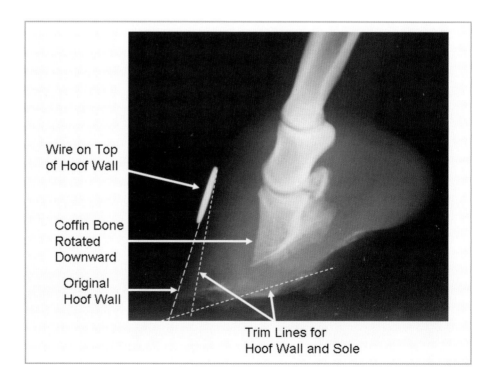

Wire on Top of Hoof Wall

Coffin Bone Rotated Downward

Original Hoof Wall

Trim Lines for Hoof Wall and Sole

Nonsteroidal anti-inflammatory drugs, such as phenylbutazone and flunixin meglumine, are often used to decrease pain and thereby improve circulation within the foot. However, pain relief may enable the donkey to move around more than is appropriate, with increased damage to the laminae. It is important to remember that donkeys are very tolerant of pain; an animal showing foot pain is most likely affected by significant disease in the feet. It is reported that 800–1,000 lb donkeys can be treated with 4 grams of phenylbutazone twice daily for 3–6 weeks if needed without any signs of drug toxicity. Doses of 1 gram daily per 500 lbs body weight can be used for 6 or more months with no obvious problems.[1]

Radiographs should be taken for most acute and all chronic laminitis cases. Lateral views are obtained of both front feet and also the hind feet if there is pain or hoof deformity of the rear hooves, as well. As mentioned, feet affected by laminitis should be trimmed as near normal as possible to approximate the ideal hoof-pastern angle of the animal based on radiographic information. It is common practice to remove toe tissue and lower the heel slightly to reestablish the normal relationship between P3 and the hoof wall, and to prevent a "hang nail" effect that could tear more laminae. The coffin bone should be supported from below with a frog support device or specialized pad. Pressure on the sole should be avoided to prevent further circulatory compromise that could add to foot damage.

Every treatment does not work in every donkey. The underlying cause(s) of laminitis must be corrected by management considerations. Weight reduction is essential to reduce stress on the feet and to improve the metabolic constitution of the donkey. Feet should be trimmed at four-week intervals at a minimum. Chronically laminitic donkeys often have recurrent foot abscesses. A donkey with laminitis is prone to recurring episodes, especially if overweight or subjected to a rapid feed change.

Summary

- The donkey and its joints are subjected to daily wear and tear during work, exercise, and even when grazing or standing still. The joints of the musculoskeletal system absorb shock, permit relatively frictionless movement, and bear the weight of a body that may weigh up to 1,200–1,500 lbs (550–650 kg).

- There are three types of joints in the body: fibrous, cartilaginous, and synovial. Fibrous joints are least likely to be afflicted with disease because they are more or less immobile. Cartilaginous joints don't have a high propensity for disease due to limited movement. Synovial joints are the most likely to suffer disease and injury because they are the most active.

- Donkeys have joint problems because they are often asked to do things they were not designed to do. Concussive force is concentrated on joints of the front legs.

- Traumatic arthritis is a diverse collection of pathological and clinical states that develop after single or repetitive episodes of trauma. Components of traumatic arthritis may include: synovitis (inflammation of the joint lining); capsulitis (inflammation of the fibrous joint capsule); strain or sprain (injury to the supporting ligaments of the joint); and fractures of bones within the joint.

- Available treatments for joint inflammation are few and may be employed as a combination of options. Rest is the most simple and often overlooked treatment. Other treatments include: anti-inflammatory medications; intra-articular corticosteroids; and various joint-specific drugs.

- Lameness is defined as an abnormality of gait caused by pain and/or restriction of movement. Most causes of lameness fall into one of the following categories: degenerative; developmental; metabolic; mechanical overload; infectious; or traumatic.

- Visual observation is the key to identifying which leg is lame. Locating the specific area involved requires two basic tools: the eyes and the hands. The skills of observation, palpation, and manipulation are employed during the exam.

- The foot is the most common site of lameness. The leg joints are another common source. Most lameness problems involve a structure at the level of or below the knee or hock.

- Diagnosis of the source of lameness may involve: physical examination; observation of gait; performance of flexion tests; palpation and manipulation; use of regional nerve blocks; ultrasonography; and radiography.

• Laminitis is an inflammatory disease of the laminar tissue, which connects the coffin bone to the inside of the hoof wall. In donkeys, it is often related to a digestive change with the resulting damage due to circulatory insufficiency to the laminae.

• Laminitis is a serious and potentially life-threatening disease of the feet. The stoic nature of donkeys might allow laminitis to advance long before showing evidence of foot pain.

• Most laminitis cases are chronic, with clinical signs only evident during an acute flare. Foot pain may be manifested as the donkey is reluctant to move even when asked as if he is "glued to the ground."

• Clinical signs of laminitis may include: misshapen hooves with diverging rings; a very stiff, short-strided gait; periodic or recurrent lameness, especially in the front feet; deviation between the coffin bones and dorsal hoof wall on radiographs; demineralization and deformity of the coffin bone; and evidence of a dropped sole.

• The key to successful laminitis treatment is early diagnosis, correction of the underlying cause, pain control, and aggressive treatment to stabilize the damage. All cases are not the same and all may not respond to a single-treatment protocol.

• Prevention of laminitis is focused on keeping donkeys from becoming obese, and on trimming the feet correctly and as frequently as necessary to maintain proper hoof health.

References

1. Personal communication with Tex Taylor, DVM, Professor of Large Animal Medicine and Surgery, Texas A and M University, College Station, TX, USA.

Reproduction

This is an overview of the practical aspects of male and female donkey reproduction. The miniature donkey is emphasized because the great majority of my experience is with miniatures, and also because there is very little information on larger donkeys at the present time. Where significant reproductive differences other than the obvious anatomical size exist between miniatures and larger donkeys, they are noted.

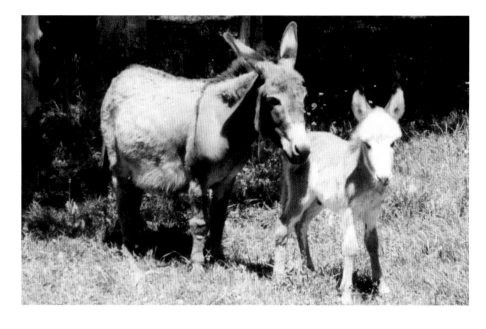

8.1 A miniature donkey jennet and her foal.

Reproductive Anatomy

Male Anatomy

The genitalia of a full-size donkey is similar to that of the full-size horse. The testes of the donkey are relatively large for the size of the animal. They are located in the scrotum and oriented vertically. The penis length of a miniature donkey is approximately 14–18 inches when fully erect, and thus a full-sized equine AV is used for semen collection. The testes and penis of larger donkeys are longer than those of comparably sized horses (figs. 8.2 A & B). Although the jack and the stallion have the same accessory sex glands, the ampulla is larger in the jack compared to the stallion.[1]

8.2 A & B Miniature donkey testes and erect penis.

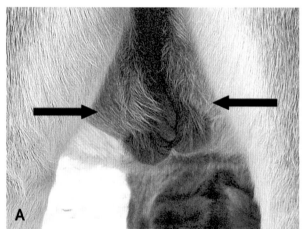
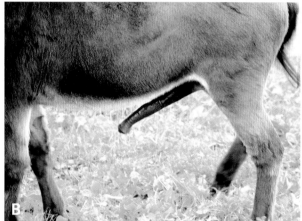

Female Anatomy

The vagina is approximately 14 inches long in the average miniature donkey. The cervix lies on the cranial vaginal floor and has a similar appearance to that of the horse with the exception that it often points upward and is usually longer than that of the mare and has a smaller diameter. A cardboard equine speculum with 6 inches removed is used for vaginal exam of the miniature donkey (fig. 8.3). It is difficult to pass pipettes or catheters through a narrow

8.3 Cardboard and plastic speculums used in any size donkeys.

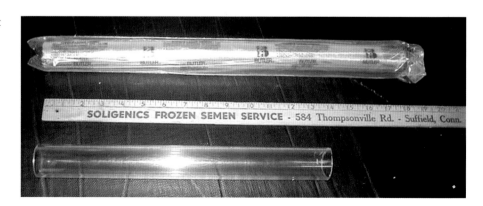

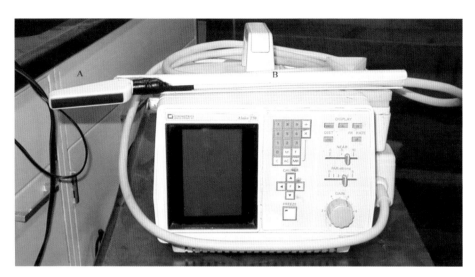

8.4 The 5 MHz Linear Probe (A) used with a 0.75 inch PVC Extension approximately 14 inches long (B) for transrectal ultrasound examinations. Note that the probe head and slot in the PVC would be covered with duct tape prior to lubrication and insertion into the rectum. The PVC extension may be left on while performing a transabdominal (through the abdomen) examination.

speculum and into the cervix because of its location in the vagina. It is best to guide these instruments with a lubricated, gloved hand in the vagina if possible. The miniature donkey uterine shape and size is similar to the standard size equine.

Transrectal (through the rectum) ultrasound examination is possible with a linear probe taped within a plastic extension (fig. 8.4). Ultrasound is useful to examine ovarian follicle size (fig. 8.5) for estimation of the opportune time to breed, and then for detection of pregnancy starting at 16 days after breeding. (For more details on ultrasound exams, see p. 109.)

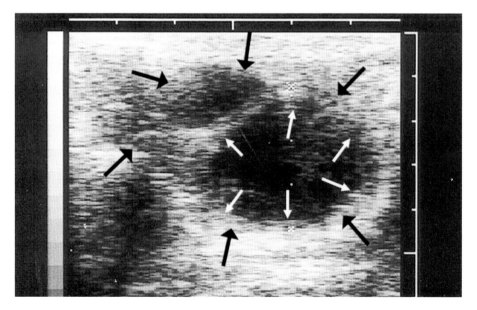

8.5 An ultrasound image of miniature donkey ovaries. Black arrows delineate border of the entire ovary. White arrows show borders of a 3.2 cm diameter ovulatory size follicle.

Reproductive Physiology and Behavior

Estrus Cycle

The estrus cycle length in donkeys is 21–28 days with the jennet sexually receptive for 5–10 days of this period. The ovulatory follicle size is similar to that in full-size equines and follicles 25–30 mm in diameter should be considered potentially ovulatory.[1,2] One miniature jennet I examined ovulated a 42 mm diameter follicle. The cervical appearance changes with the stage of the estrus cycle, relaxing during estrus, which is accompanied with an increase in vaginal mucous secretions. Jennets may cycle throughout the winter.

Reproductive Behavior

A jennet often shows her first heat at 8–12 months of age. Female receptivity is evidenced by the jennet backing up to the jack and making jawing motions with the mouth (figs. 8.6 A & B). Jennets in estrus will kick a jack in the chest (and the face if the jack is not careful) for several minutes when receptive (fig. 8.7). This behavior is required for the jack to achieve full erection. Receptive jennets also squat, wink the vulva, and urinate in the presence of the jack. A receptive jennet may also raise her tail when approached by a jack. Jennets mount each other on occasion, with the estrus jennet on the bottom. Some jennets do not show receptivity when there is no jack present, when nursing a foal, or when another female interferes with the advances of the jack.

8.6 A & B The jawing behavior exhibited by a jennet in heat when being mounted by a jack.

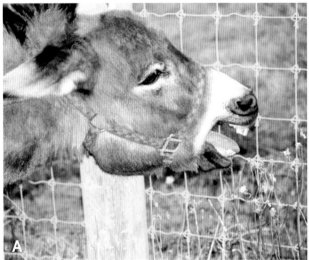
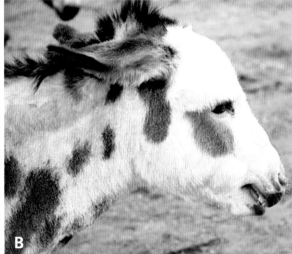

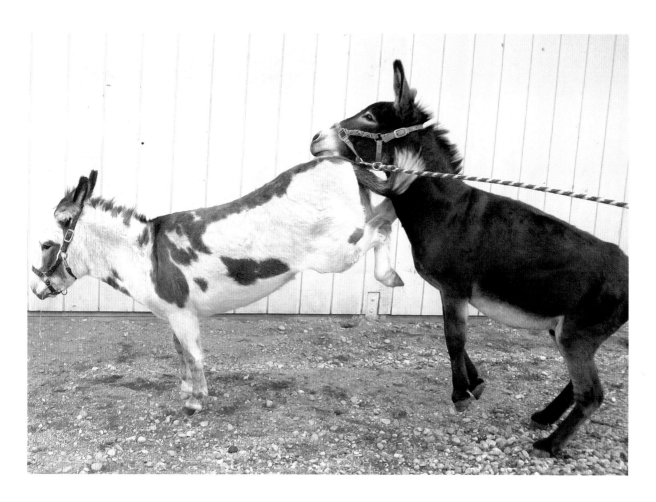

A jack pursues the jennet in estrus, sometimes very aggressively, especially when first introduced. He may bite the neck, back, and hind legs and
even draw blood. As a consequence, some jacks have to wear a breeding
muzzle to avoid injury to the jennet. Jacks usually calm down after a short
time (15–30 minutes) and then the muzzle may be removed. It is easy to
teach most jacks to mount without biting the jennet by using a chain lead
shank over the nose. Vigorous jerking motions on the chain along with verbal
commands usually result in a quick learning process for the jack. Donkeys are
intelligent animals and respond well to consistent, firm training methods.

A jennet may back up to the jack after having ovulated, but he may not
mount her if he has recently bred her (within a few hours) or has been collected for artificial insemination. Normally, a jack will mount a jennet a few times
before becoming fully erect, and some jacks are relatively slow to achieve
erection (10–15 minutes) when compared to horses. It is common for multi-

8.7 A jennet in heat kicking
the approaching jack.

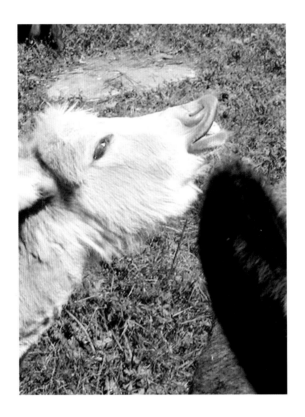

8.8 A juvenile miniature donkey exhibiting flehmen-reaction behavior when approaching a jennet in heat.

ple mounts to be required along with some periods of inactivity at a short distance from the jennet before the jack achieves a full erection and completes a breeding. In my opinion, there is no correlation between time to achieve full erection or degree of aggressive breeding behavior and fertility. The jack responds to a jennet's jawing behavior with vocalization and flehmen (fig. 8.8). Some jacks are timid and will not breed when new people are present.

Field Breeding

Jack owners most commonly use field breeding by turning one jack out with as many as 10 jennets. The jack selects the most receptive jennet to breed by checking the herd's manure for pheromones (chemical olfactory messengers) that may be involved in estrus detection. Receptive jennets may also approach a breeding pair to attract the jack.

Hand Breeding

Controlled, hand or "appointment" breeding allows for recording of exact breeding dates. The breeding cycle may be coordinated with serial transrectal ultrasound examinations of the ovaries to determine the time of ovulation and the best time to breed. Jacks may be overly aggressive or timid when first training them to mount in controlled situations; however, they are fast learners. Estrus synchronization protocols useful in horses seem to be effective in the donkey. If hand breeding is used, it is suggested that the jennet be bred the second day of heat (estrus) and then at 48-hour intervals until the end of standing heat.[3]

Artificial Insemination

Artificial insemination (AI) is possible on the farm or with transported fresh, cooled semen. Jacks are easy to train for collection although this technique is not currently used on a widespread basis. Miniature donkey semen is very concentrated (see p. 122 for detailed discussion) and in general has good fertility. Donkey semen can be handled similarly to that of the stallion, and skim milk extenders seem to be useful for keeping sperm alive during transport in artificial insemination programs.[4] French workers have published freezing protocols for donkey semen.[5]

Ultrasound Examination of the Female Reproductive Tract

This section describes the technique for examination of the female donkey reproductive tract. The reproductive exam is not difficult for a veterinarian to perform once some basic landmarks and procedures are learned. It is also safe for the animal, in my opinion. The techniques described here are useful for estimating stage of estrus, determining the optimum time for artificial insemination or hand breeding, deciding to stop breeding after ovulation of a follicle has occurred, or determining the pregnancy status of a particular animal.

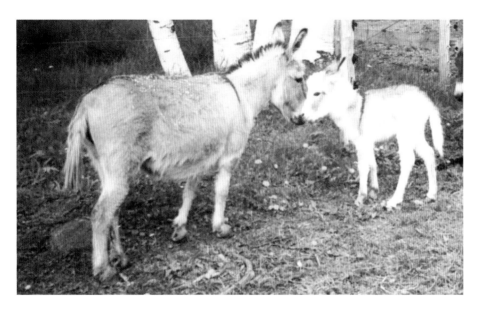

8.9 The result of successful field or hand breeding, or AI: a jennet and her foal.

A veterinarian can tell the stage of pregnancy accurately and early on by using commonly available ultrasound equipment. A 5 MHz linear probe is adequate for such examinations (see fig. 8.4, p. 105). Transrectal and transabdominal techniques are possible and well tolerated by most jennets without sedation. During estrus, the examiner can follow follicles as they mature and regress, and also identify the *corpus hemorrhagicum* (blood-filled follicle following ovulation) and the *corpus luteum* (stage of development of a follicle following ovulation and blood filling that secretes hormones to maintain conception if it occurs) produced successively on the ovary at the ovulation site.

Transrectal examination can detect pregnancy as early as 16 days after breeding. I am currently developing tables for miniature donkeys to relate the diameter of the *conceptus* (embryo) to the stage of pregnancy. The fetal heartbeat may be seen at approximately 25 days of pregnancy. Transabdominal examinations are easily performed after 70–80 days in miniature donkeys (see fig. 8.17, p. 116) yet it is more difficult to estimate stage of pregnancy after 90 days. I have pending pregnancy ultrasound and reproductive cycle studies that aim to refine the diagnostic accuracy for miniatures.

Suggested Reading

• Purdy, SR. "Reproduction in Miniature Donkeys." *Veterinary Care of Donkeys*. Matthews, NS, and Taylor, TS (Eds.). International Veterinary Information Service, Ithaca, NY (www.ivis.org).

Equipment Setup

Animal Handling

One of the keys to performing a safe and thorough ultrasound examination is in the handling of the animal. Some basic handling rules must be followed since donkeys do not like to be hurried. What has erroneously been referred to as stubbornness is actually caution and a donkey's typical evaluation process. Donkeys will tolerate a non-painful procedure if the people involved are patient in their approach. Donkeys tend to stop or back up, and so should be offered time to look the situation over rather than being pushed or lifted, which just frustrates and tires the humans and frightens the animals. Donkeys can sometimes be backed into a convenient location to perform an examination.

Most examinations are performed in a chute arrangement with the animal tied to the front end with a halter and lead rope (fig. 8.10). One excellent

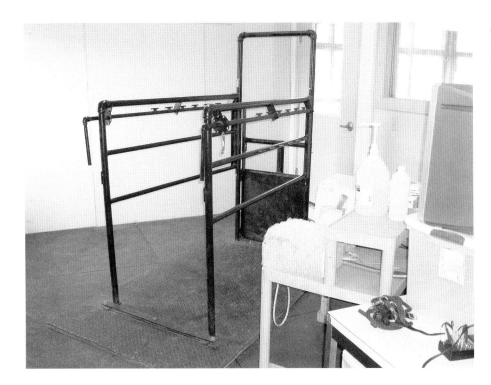

8.10 A chute setup for performing ultrasound examinations.

motivator to entice a donkey to enter the chute is to offer a dish of sweet feed at the front end. A donkey's first trip in may take a while, but subsequent entry is usually faster with the food incentive present. Reproductive exams do not take much time so eating keeps the animal occupied and quiet. There may be trouble leading one animal into the examination chute from a holding pen of many as all will try to get to the food! Many exams are performed without a chute by standing a haltered animal next to a solid wall or tying her to a solid object. An assistant can also position a donkey with its rear end adjacent to a stall door and the ultrasound equipment safely located just outside. Food distraction also works well with these methods.

The internal anatomy of the female reproductive tract of the donkey, miniature included, is comparable to that of a 1,000 lb horse in regards to size of the uterus, ovaries, and length of the tract. This must be kept in mind when performing transrectal examinations so as not to mistakenly search for the ovaries at a location based on scaling down the size of the animal. Examinations should be performed in a quiet, but not necessarily isolated, location since donkeys are comforted by the presence of other animals within close proximity. It is helpful if other animals are located in an adjacent pen or stall. Good lighting encourages the animals to enter the proper location, but it is also useful to be able to reduce light intensity to allow for easy viewing of the ultrasound screen. The machine can be placed on a portable cart or hay bales in close proximity for ease of viewing by the operator and operation of machine controls, such as those for freezing the picture for measuring or to capture it as a digital or printed image.

Examination Techniques

Transrectal Examinations

Transrectal examination of the miniature donkey uterus and ovaries is most often performed by attaching a 5 MHz ultrasound probe to a ¾ inch diameter, slotted PVC extension arm of approximately 14 inches in length (fig. 8.11). This is necessary because size limitations constrain most veterinarians from introducing hand and arm fully into the rectum as is possible in the full-size equine. A gloved and lubricated hand is first used to evacuate manure with three fingers just inside the anus. Then, 120 ml of water-soluble lubricant is gently infused through the anus into the rectum using a catheter tip syringe. This aids in introducing the probe safely into the proper position for the examination, and it provides good contact between the probe and the rectal wall for improved imaging of the uterus and ovaries. The rectum does not have to be completely evacuated for the exam.

8.11 An extended ultrasound probe being inserted into the rectum for examination.

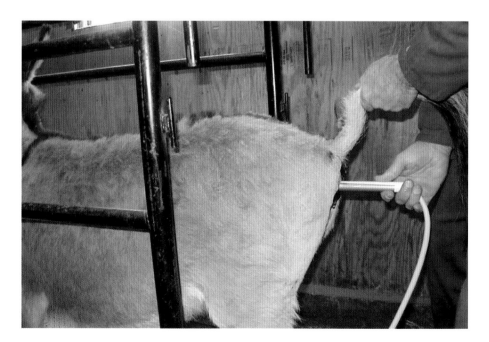

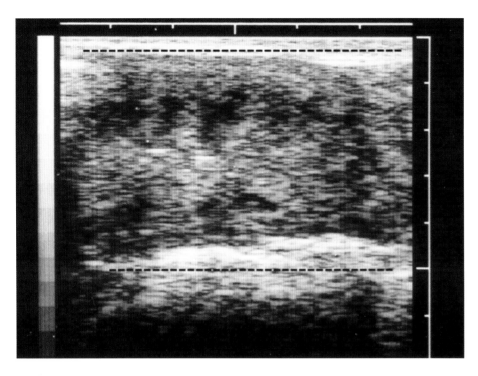

8.12 A longitudinal, transrectal ultrasound image of the uterine body of a donkey during estrus. Note anechoic (black) mottling representative of edema in the uterine lining during estrus. Scale: 10 mm per division.

In larger donkeys whose rectums are able to safely accommodate the passage of the examiner's hand and the probe, no extensor arm is needed. Emptying the rectum and use of copious amounts of lubricant are necessary in larger donkeys. If resistance is encountered or feces interfere with transmission and reception of the ultrasound waves when slowly advancing the probe in a miniature or small donkey, manure should be removed—an enema of 300 ml warm, soapy water can be administered. The animal is returned to the holding area, and the exam is recommenced after the animal evacuates the manure. This is necessary for less than 10% of transrectal exams. The ultrasound probe is further lubricated with external application of lubricant before introduction into the rectum.

The probe is initially advanced through the anal sphincter in a 45-degree upward direction to allow for the tilt of the donkey pelvis. At 4–6 inches inside the rectum, the urinary bladder is visualized at the 6 o'clock (bottom) position, a convenient landmark to locate and visualize the uterus, which is found just in front of the bladder. The body of the Y-shaped uterus is seen as a linear structure as the probe is advanced. A cross-sectional view of the uterine horns is obtained as the probe is advanced and rotated to the 5 and 7 o'clock positions at approximately 12–14 inches in from the anus (fig. 8.12).

The probe may have to be moved gently in and out or rotated slightly to find the right and left horns for examination. Once the smallest diameter of the respective horn is found, the probe is rotated to either the 3 or 9 o'clock positions at that depth of insertion to locate the ovary. Again slight rotation, insertion, or withdrawal of the probe may facilitate viewing of each entire ovary (figs. 8.13 A & B).

At times, examination of one side or the other may not be possible due to the presence of manure between the probe and the rectal wall. The probe may be used to gently rotate the manure out of the way for a clearer view. On some occasions, the ovaries just cannot be found or the uterus cannot be fully examined due to interference from intestine moving between the rectum and the reproductive organs. It is best to stop the exam and try another time. If any size donkey strains at any time during the examination procedure, termi-

8.13 A & B Ultrasound views of both ovaries of a donkey during estrus. Scales are 10 mm per division. Note multiple follicles (large, black areas) in the left image and the large, dominant follicle in the right image.

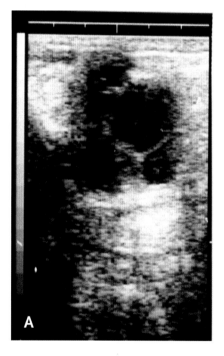
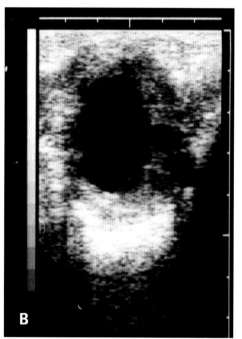

nate the exam immediately. Damage to the rectum is a slight risk with an ultrasound exam, and careful and slow examination minimizes this possibility.

Ultrasound pregnancy examinations are performed using either a transrectal or transabdominal technique depending on the gestational age of the fetus. The *conceptus* may be found using the transrectal technique from as

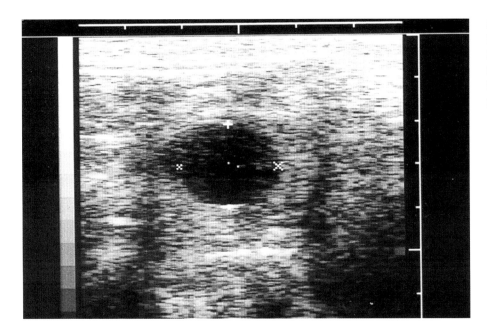

8.14 An 18-day pregnancy in a miniature donkey. The black circle represents the area of embryonic fluid associated with the pregnancy.

early as 16 days of pregnancy (fig. 8.14), at which time it is usually located in the 6 o'clock position just forward of the urinary bladder. The distance of probe or hand insertion depends on the amount of filling of the bladder. The *conceptus* is generally identified between the 5 and 7 o'clock positions as pregnancy progresses. The depth of probe penetration in miniature or small donkeys varies with age of the jennet; multiparous (having had mul-

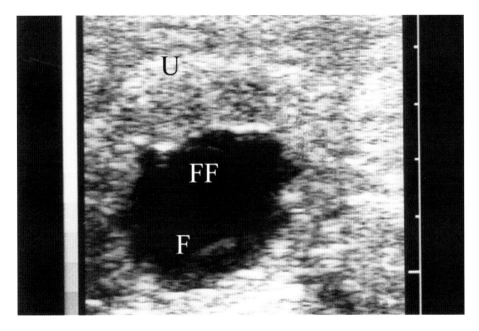

8.15 A 37-day pregnancy. F = fetus; FF = fetal fluids; U = uterine wall.

tiple offspring) females usually require a deeper reach. For example, a 37-day pregnancy (fig. 8.15) may be found as far as 15 inches forward of the anus. The extended probe may have to be deviated fully downward at the front end to visualize the fetus. The donkey fetal heartbeat, first seen at approximately 25 days, appears as an on-and-off flicker of fluid density as the heart fills and contracts.

The maximum gestational age at which the miniature donkey fetus may be found using the transrectal technique is still under investigation. It is expected to vary based on the number of previous foals of the jennet, and on the body type of the animal. There is usually a time period in most species when the pregnant uterine horn is drawn down over the brim of the pelvis and into the lower abdomen by the weight of the fetus, pulling the fetus out of range for ultrasound detection. However, fetal fluids and the placenta may be visualized at a later stage without being able to visualize the actual fetus.

Transabdominal Examinations

At approximately 70–80 days of gestation, the miniature donkey fetus may be visualized using the transabdominal technique near the midline of the rear portion of the abdomen (figs. 8.16 and 8.17). No information is currently

8.16 A 5 MHz linear probe applied to the caudoventral abdomen of a miniature donkey for performance of transabdominal ultrasound uterine examination at 70–80 days of pregnancy and beyond.

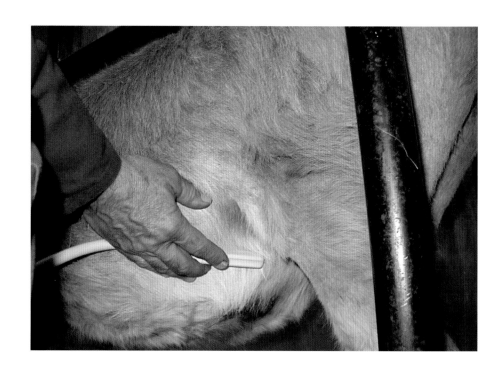

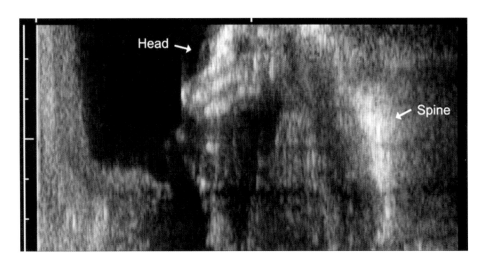

8.17 An ultrasound image of a 72-day miniature donkey fetus.

available for larger donkeys. As in the transrectal technique, a coupling medium is needed for good transmission and reception of the ultrasound waves between the probe and the tissue to which it is applied. Water-soluble methylcellulose lubricant or alcohol serves this function by liberal application to the donkey's abdomen. Abdominal hair does not have to be clipped, and I have found that alcohol tends to give a clearer picture than gel. Application of additional alcohol or gel to the probe and skin during the exam is likely to be needed to maintain the best picture quality.

As pregnancy progresses, there is relatively less fluid and more soft tissue density seen when examining the fetus (fig. 8.18). Fetal movement is consistently seen 90% of the time. If a few minutes are allowed beyond the initial look, fetal movement is usually seen, characterized by jerking or twitching. This movement is different from that of move-

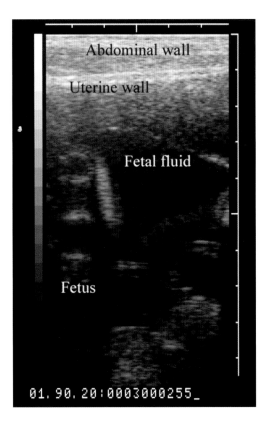

8.18 An ultrasound image of a 255-day miniature donkey fetus.

Suggested Reading

• Purdy, SR. "Ultrasound Examination of the Reproductive Tract in Female Miniature Donkeys." *Veterinary Care of Donkeys*. Matthews, NS, and Taylor, TS (Eds.). International Veterinary Information Service, Ithaca, NY (www.ivis.org).

ment of digestive organs and their contents. If in doubt, the discovery of the fetal heartbeat finalizes the diagnosis. In the last trimester of pregnancy, the fetal heartbeat is usually found on the ventral abdomen adjacent to the umbilicus. Currently, I am performing examinations on pregnant miniature donkeys at various stages of gestation to obtain detailed information on the appearance of the fetus throughout gestation.

Artificial Insemination for Miniature Donkeys

Artificial insemination is a viable technique for use in ponies, miniature horses, and miniature donkeys. Standard equine equipment may be used to collect, evaluate, transport, and inseminate semen. Limited experience exists with fresh cooled semen and immediate post-collection insemination in donkeys.

Semen Collection

Standard equine collection equipment can be used in donkeys of all sizes, including miniature donkeys. I have exclusively used the 16-inch Missouri Artificial Vagina (AV), which is available from various sources (fig. 8.19 A). Collection may also be performed with the Roanoke AV (Roanoke AI Laboratories, Roanoke, VA, 540-774-0676 or www.roanokeai.com).

It is easy to train a jack for semen collection, even one that is only used to field breeding, by using a jump jennet that is in estrus. Proper handling is important—the handlers and collector must be patient and allow for the normal, cautious behavior of donkeys when confronted with new situations. As always, grain is an excellent motivator to entice a donkey into an unfamiliar area. The collection process with donkeys is different from horses due to the different reproductive behavior of the donkey. A jack may take as long as 30 minutes to achieve a full erection (see fig. 8.2 B, p. 104). As the jack approaches a jennet in estrus, she will "jaw" (open and close her mouth) (see figs. 8.6 A & B, p. 106). The jack should not be allowed to bite the jennet, or to

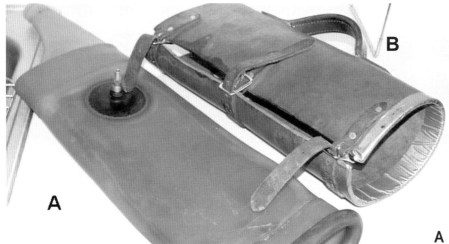

8.19 A A full-size Missouri Artificial Vagina (AV) used to collect miniature donkey jacks.
A = liner;
B = leather cover/carrier.

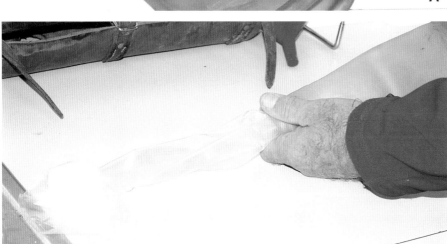

8.19 B Inserting the disposable, sterile AV liner into the water-filled AV liner.

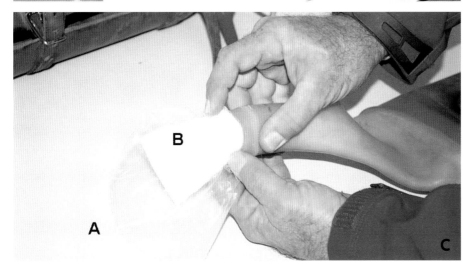

8.19 C Fixing the gel filter in place.
A = collection end of disposable, sterile, plastic AV liner;
B = inline semen gel filter.

8.19 D An insulated mug with a thermometer inserted being filled with water at the proper temperature to fill the rubber AV liner.

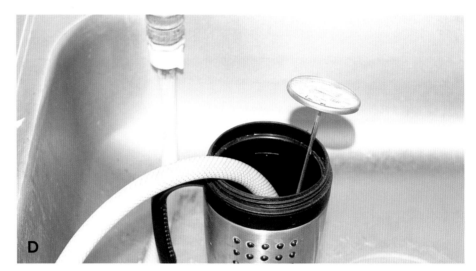

8.19 E Filling the rubber AV Liner by pouring 115°F water into a funnel attached to the liner.

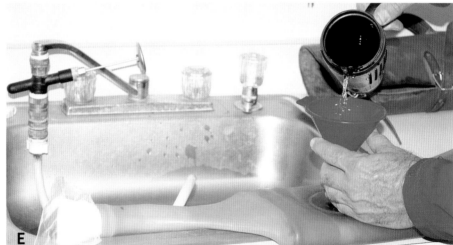

8.19 F Carrying the assembled AV.

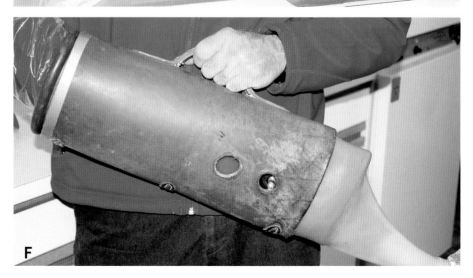

stay on her back until he has achieved a full erection. He should be handled with a chain lead shank over the nose when first training him for collection to make him pay attention to the handler. The chain soon becomes unnecessary with most jacks as they readily take to the collection procedure.

In this description of collection, the 16-inch Missouri AV is used, along with a sterile disposable liner with attached gel filter. The jack initially teases the jennet to verify that she is in a strong, standing heat. Note that she will kick the jack in the chest on approach and that this seems to be necessary for him to achieve an erection. The jack is kept in sight of the jennet, but not in close physical contact while the AV is prepared. A disposable liner with an in-line gel filter is inserted into the apparatus and taped over the opening for the penis (figs. 8.19 B & C). The rubber AV liner is filled with tap water at a temperature of approximately 115°F. Temperature may be verified by filling a small insulated, plastic thermos bottle or cup with water and measuring with a thermometer (fig. 8.19 D). The AV liner is completely filled, all air expelled, and then the leather cover is placed over it (fig. 8.19 E). Non-spermicidal, sterile lubricant is applied to a long, plastic OB sleeve on the collector's arm, which is inserted into the AV to carry it and help maintain water temperature (fig. 8.19 F), an important feature in cold weather collections.

The jennet may be tied in a corner or be controlled by a handler in an

8.20 Teasing the non-erect jack under handler's control until he achieves a full erection.

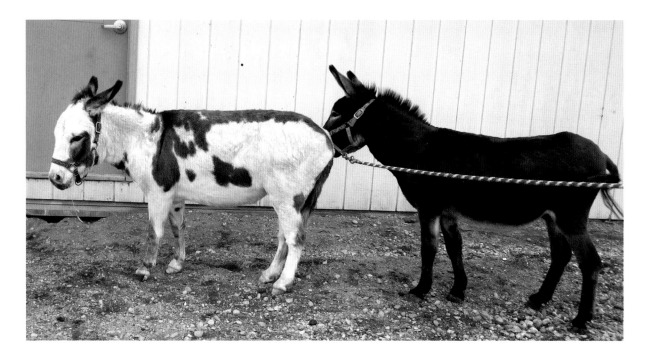

8.21 Directing the erect jack penis into a Missouri AV after the jack has mounted the receptive jennet.

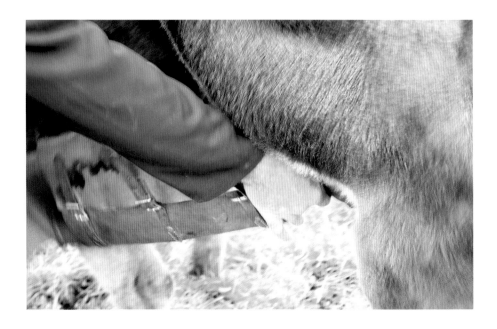

aisle that provides good footing for both donkeys. The jack handler should tease the jack until he is fully erect (fig. 8.20). Only then should he be allowed to mount and stay on the jennet. It is helpful to learn the individual breeding characteristics of the animals involved. After the fully erect jack is allowed to mount, the collector handling the AV quickly directs the jack's penis into the AV (fig. 8.21). The other hand is placed at the base of the penis to feel for ejaculation. The collector should strip the penis into the AV after ejaculation when the jack dismounts.

The next procedures are performed in rapid succession to preserve the maximum amount of viable semen. Water is drained from the AV to allow collected semen to drain through the filter and into the collection receptacle tip, which is opened with scissors. Semen is drawn into a preheated (stored in a 100°F incubator), all-plastic syringe, and all syringes should remain in an incubator until used for insemination. The collected dose may be split if needed for more than one jennet, depending on the semen characteristics of the collected jack. Other collection methods are under investigation, including use of a phantom jennet and ground collection without a jennet or phantom.

Semen Evaluation

Semen can be collected for evaluation after hand-breeding, natural cover by grasping the jack penis immediately after dismount and letting semen drip into a warmed plastic tube. The evaluation procedures for donkeys used by the author are those used for horses. Parameters to evaluate include:

- Semen volume (mL)
- Sperm concentration (sperm x 106 per mL)
- Progressive motility (%)
- Morphology (form or shape) of sperm (%)
- Total number useful sperm in the ejaculate (x106)

Semen volume is measured after removing it from the AV collection reservoir tip with the plastic syringes. Sperm concentration may be measured inexpensively using the Unopette® WBC and hemocytometer method. Motility and morphology are determined using a standard microscope, and morphology is further evaluated using a nigrosin-eosin stain, which demonstrates which sperm are alive and which are dead. The total number of useful sperm in the ejaculate is determined by multiplying the first four parameters together. At the present time, I have not determined the minimal number of sperm to be used in donkey insemination. It seems reasonable to use the numbers recommended for horses until further studies have been completed.

Semen collected from miniature donkeys by myself and Brian Ramsey, DVM, of Tyler, Texas, has been evaluated and characteristics are tabulated in Table 1 with comparisons shown to full-size and miniature horses. (Miniature horse values are courtesy of Ron Emond, DVM, Bridgewater, Connecticut.)

Miniature Donkeys	Average	Range	Horse Normals	Miniature Horse Normals
Semen Volume (mL)	25–50	21–115	60–80	20–45
Progressive Motility (%)	80–90	65–90	70–90	>75
Sperm Concentration (x 10^6)	200–500	75–877	60–150	250–350
Normal Morphology (%)	80–90	69–92	70–90	Similar
Useful Sperm per Ejaculate (x 10^6)	5,000–11,000	3,307–18,000	Less	6,000–10,000

Table 1 Miniature donkey semen characteristics (16 animals).

Summary of miniature donkey semen parameter data as compared to horses:

- Volume is lower than full-sized horses.
- Motility is comparable to horses.
- Sperm concentration is generally higher than horses.
- Total number of useful sperm is generally higher per ejaculate.

In general, mini-donkey semen has qualities on par or better than horse semen collected in a similar fashion.

Shipping Fresh Cooled Semen

Limited experience and data are available with regard to the efficacy of shipping miniature donkey semen; however, the experiences of myself and Dr. Ramsey indicate that it can be done. More work is needed to establish standard protocols. Scarcity of data is largely due to reluctance of donkey owners, particularly stud owners, to use artificial insemination as a breeding technique. This is fairly normal for any animal species when a novel reproductive technique is first introduced.

Semen shipping containers used with success are the Equitainer® (Hamilton Thorne Research, Inc., South Hamilton, MA, www.equitainer.com/home) and the Equine Express II (Exodus Breeders Supply, York, PA, www.exodusbreeders.com). Semen extenders in current use contain antibiotics and nutrients to help maintain semen viability. Examples include Kenney's with ticarcillin or EZ Mixin® containing amikacin, ticarcillin, polymixin B, and potassium penicillin.

Management of the Female

The goal for AI when using transported semen is to breed only once per cycle. If a stud is available to tease the female, the process is easier since he helps determine the timing for semen to be ordered from the stud owner. If a stud is not locally available, the timing of insemination may be selected by using hormonal control with a prostaglandin injection to induce estrus, as is done in the mare. Ultrasound evaluation of the ovaries and uterus and the changes associated with estrus and ovulation are also followed with transrectal ultrasound (see p. 112). A vaginal speculum exam tracks cervical changes as in the mare and this procedure corroborates information gained from the transrectal ultrasound exam. The use of HCG (human chorionic gonadotropin) to induce ovulation in donkeys is under investigation.

Artificial Insemination Technique

The technique of artificial insemination is similar in all equine species. Semen is stored in an incubator for on-farm insemination or in the cooled semen transport container until it is ready to be used. The jennet's tail is wrapped or covered with a taped on, inverted plastic sleeve for cleanliness, and the tail is tied out of the way. Her vulva and the surrounding area are cleaned with soap and water followed by thorough rinsing to prevent soap toxicity to sperm, and then allowed to dry. A long-sleeved, sterile glove, a plastic pipette, non-spermicidal lubricant, and an all-plastic syringe are used for insemination. The inseminator's gloved and lubricated hand carries the sterile pipette into the vagina. One finger is inserted into the cervix and the pipette is passed into the uterine body, aiming slightly toward the horn on the side of the ovary with the largest follicle. The semen-filled syringe(s) is attached to the pipette to deliver semen with a gentle push. The cervix is "feathered" with a finger (touched lightly with an up-and-down motion) before withdrawing the gloved hand from the vagina. If the jennet's vagina is too small to insert a hand, the technique becomes more difficult to perform; it can be challenging to pass a pipette into a donkey cervix, which tends to be located on the floor of the vagina, pointing slightly upward. Alternate techniques for insemination are being researched, including use of cervical forceps to hold the cervix rigidly in position, and the use of a fiberoptic endoscope.

Suggested Reading

- Purdy, SR. "Ultrasound Examination of the Female Miniature Donkey." *New England Journal of Large Animal Health*. 2002; 2(2):75-78.

- Matthews, NS, and Taylor, TS (Eds.). "Artificial Insemination for Miniature Donkeys." *Veterinary Care of Donkeys*. International Veterinary Information Service, Ithaca, NY (www.ivis.org).

Pregnancy Determination

Transrectal ultrasound can be safely and accurately performed at 16-plus days to visualize the *conceptus*. Failure of a jennet to return to estrus only means that a *corpus luteum* is present and not necessarily that conception has occurred. Behavioral estrus may not be possible to observe unless a stud is available for teasing. Hormone analyses using estrone sulfate or pregnant mare serum gonadotropin (PMSG) have not been used extensively in donkeys.

Suggested Websites

Websites with good references concerning AI in horses:

- Hamilton Research, Inc. (www.equitainer.com/home)
- Roanoke AI Laboratories (www.roanokeai.com)
- Exodus Breeders Supply (www.exodusbreeders.com)
- Select Breeders Services (www.selectbreeders.com)

Frozen Semen

Presently, limited data and experience are available regarding the use of frozen semen in donkeys. Miniature donkey semen can be frozen and thawed successfully (Purdy/Ballard 2001), with approximately 30% motility following thawing; as yet, I have no experience using frozen semen for donkey AI. This technique has the potential benefit of sharing genetic material around the world. More work is needed to explore this technique and to evaluate its effectiveness.

Castration

Castration is performed on donkeys to neuter animals not intended for breeding purposes. This procedure can be performed on young donkeys at least 6 months of age or older and should only be performed by a competent, qualified veterinarian under clean environmental conditions.

The scrotal blood vessels are relatively larger and the scrotal skin is thicker than in the horse. Consequently, donkeys are more prone to bleeding during this surgical procedure. I recommend ligation of the vascular cord with suture material along with the use of hemostats instead of an emasculator for castration.

Preparation for Anesthesia

Castration may be safely performed in a barn environment and does not always require a sterile surgical room. Select a clean, well lit, and quiet environment for the surgery and for safe recovery from anesthesia. The anesthetic protocol used is relatively short-acting, so all materials necessary for the procedure should be assembled in advance.

Pre-Anesthetic Physical Examination

A brief physical examination is suggested prior to surgery. Parameters checked include: auscultation (listening with a stethoscope) of the heart, lungs, trachea, and intestinal tract; evaluation of mucous membrane color and hydration status; and location and palpation of both testicles. Ideally, the tetanus immunization status of the donkey should be up to date prior to surgery. If not, then tetanus toxoid should be administered immediately.

Induction of Anesthesia

The anesthetic combination used for the castration surgery is a mixture of three commonly used large animal drugs. One method for induction of anesthesia is to sedate with xylazine (1.1 mg/kg, IV) and then induce general anesthesia with ketamine (2.2 mg/kg, IV) after 3–5 minutes. If insufficient sedation is obtained, as evidenced by the jack responding to a tap on the forehead, additional sedative should be given IV before administering the general anesthetic. Addition of butorphanol (0.01–0.02 mg/kg, IV) or diazepam (0.0.03 mg/kg, IV) increases the level of sedation and muscle relaxation. Onset of anesthesia usually occurs 2–3 minutes after ketamine injection. Do not feel rushed to get the animal down as stimulation prolongs or delays the induction period.

Sedation followed by injectable general anesthesia provides around 15–20 minutes of anesthesia in most donkeys. Miniature donkeys seem refractory to these drug dosages even for a short procedure, showing muscle rigidity and excitatory effects.[6] I have achieved satisfactory results in miniature donkeys by increasing the dose rates of the xylazine, butorphanol, and ketamine combination above by 25%.

If additional anesthetic is needed during the procedure it may be administered intravenously in the jugular vein or medial saphenous vein of the leg at half the original dose, with the sedative and anesthetic drugs combined in the same syringe.

Surgery

The upper leg is tied up and away from the body to expose the surgery site. An incision is made with a scalpel through the skin to expose the lower testicle, which is pulled out of the incision and the vascular cord is isolated by bluntly stripping away the fat associated with it. The attachment of the *cremaster muscle* is broken with finger pressure where it joins the testicle. Fat that prolapses out of the incision should be removed with blunt finger and gauze pad dissection. I use three clamps and two ties for the vascular cord of each testicle. I do not recommend the use of an emasculator instrument on miniature donkeys, although others use it with success. I will use it on large-size donkeys, but I also always use one clamp and one tie above the instrument to assure that any bleeding only originates from minor scrotal vessels rather than the large vascular cord. After removing the testicle and ensuring that no hemorrhage is present, the remaining vascular stump is pushed back into the incision. The upper testicle is removed in a similar fashion. It is also important to stretch the skin incisions with the fingers after all instruments have been removed—this keeps them open for drainage of blood or serum. At this time any additional fat prolapsed through the incision is removed.

Recovery from Anesthesia

Donkeys generally recover from anesthesia without excitement if good analgesia has been provided. Recovery should be supervised and uncommonly, it may be necessary to provide additional oxygen via a tube into the nose or larynx. Breathing difficulty is often relieved simply by extending the donkey's head and neck. Recovery times from most anesthetics in donkeys are slower than in horses. Miniature donkeys may recover more rapidly than larger donkeys.

Roll the animal into a sternal position and make sure there is a good air flow pathway. Recovery usually takes up to 20 minutes before the animal is standing up. Often the donkey is more stable in the front end before the rear end works as efficiently. Donkeys generally do not stand up until fully recovered, unlike the horse, which may make attempts to stand before being fully ready. It is also not unusual for donkeys to stand up, hind end first, while balancing on a front knee like a cow.[7] As he attempts to rise, holding on to the base of his tail helps to stabilize the donkey. He should be monitored closely until fully recovered and able to walk on his own.

Food should be withheld for an hour after recovery since sedatives and general anesthetics decrease intestinal activity. Obstruction of the esophagus (choke) can occur if donkeys try to eat immediately following anesthesia.[8]

Post-Operative Care

Following recovery from surgery, the donkey should be kept quiet and not have to deal with herd competitors for the rest of that day and night. Confinement in a box stall is recommended to minimize movement and associated bleeding; the next morning, he should be turned out for exercise. The day after surgery, the donkey should act completely normal in his appetite and attitude. If not, call your veterinarian immediately.

Animals that do not move much voluntarily should be hand walked for 15 minutes, twice daily for the first 5–7 days after surgery—this ensures continued drainage of fluid from the incisions and limits swelling that might obscure drainage. The new gelding may still have a desire to mount jennets for weeks to months; this behavior may even continue for years depending on the age at castration and the inherent aggressiveness of the animal involved. Usually, it is safe to turn him back out with females after 4 weeks without worrying about impregnation of a jennet in the herd. His behavior may not significantly change, but without testicles or sperm, it is unlikely for him to get jennets pregnant.

Summary

- The reproductive anatomy of the male donkey is similar to that of the standard horse. The same applies for the female, including the size of the reproductive tract.

- Female donkeys have a 21–28 day estrus cycle with obvious behavioral signs of receptivity when a jack is present.

- Lactation may stop a donkey from cycling while other females (related or not) may interfere with displays of sexual receptivity and breeding.

- Field and hand breeding are used in donkeys.

- Transrectal and transabdominal ultrasound are safe, effective methods for reproductive examinations.

- It is not difficult for a veterinarian familiar with ultrasound reproductive examinations to accomplish ultrasound successfully. Confidence level and accuracy increase rapidly with the number of examinations performed. Useful information that improves reproductive efficiency is easily obtained using basic ultrasound equipment.

- Artificial insemination (AI) is a viable technique, although it is not widely accepted by donkey owners at this time.

- Standard equine equipment may be used to collect, evaluate, transport, and inseminate semen in donkeys. Limited experience exists with fresh-cooled and immediate post-collection semen insemination. AI with frozen semen has the potential to be a valuable breeding technique.

- Timing of insemination for females may be successfully managed using serial ultrasound exams and hormonal control with prostaglandin and HCG injections.

- Castration is performed on donkeys to neuter animals not intended for breeding purposes. This procedure can be done on young donkeys at least 6 months of age or older and should only be performed by a competent, qualified veterinarian under clean environmental conditions.

- Castration may be safely performed in a barn environment and does not always require a sterile surgical room. The anesthetic protocol used is relatively short-acting, so all materials necessary for the procedure should be assembled in advance.

- Donkeys generally recover from anesthesia without excitement if good analgesia has been provided. Recovery should be supervised, and uncommonly it may be necessary to provide additional oxygen via a tube into the nose or larynx.

- Following recovery from castration surgery, the donkey should be kept quiet and not have to deal with herd competitors for the rest of that day and night. Confinement in a box stall is recommended to minimize movement and associated bleeding; the next morning, he should be turned out for exercise. The day after surgery, the donkey should act completely normal in his appetite and attitude.

References

1. Pugh, DG. "Donkey Reproduction." Proceedings of the Annual Convention of the AAEP. 2002; 113–114.

2. Vandeplassche, GM, et al. "Behavior, Follicular and Gonadotropin Changes During the Estrus Cycle in Donkeys." *Theriogenology.* 1981; 7:169–174.

3. Ferlding, D. "Reproductive Characteristics of the Jenny Donkey—Equus assinus: a review." *Tropical Animal Health Production.* 1988; 20:161–166.

4. Singhui, NM. "Studies on Artificial Insemination in Equines." *International Journal of Animal Research.* 1990; 11:99–104.

5. Trineche, A, et al. "A Procedure for Poitou Jackass Sperm Cryopreservation." *Theriogenology.* 1998; 50:793–806.

6. Matthews, NS, Van Dijk, P. "Anesthesia and Analgesia for Donkeys." *Veterinary Care for Donkeys.* International Veterinary Information Service, Ithaca, NY (www.ivis.org) 2004.

7. See note 1 above.

8. See note 1 above.

Pregnancy, Neonatology, and Lactation

Monitoring Pregnancy

Gestational length in the donkey is approximately 12–13 months with some researchers reporting average length of 372–374 days.[1] Pregnancy confirmation using standard ultrasound equipment can begin at 16 days following breeding with additional ultrasounds beginning at 25–28 days of gestation. By this time, based on an average estrus cycle of 28 days, the jennet should either be pregnant or have returned to estrus. If she had been confirmed pregnant with an embryo at around 16 days yet she is neither in estrus nor pregnant at 28 days, then the *conceptus* has undergone early embryonic death. This is not as dire an occurrence as it sounds as it is advantageous for bad embryos to die early so that the jennet may be rebred.

Rebreeding is indicated depending on time of the year and the number of previous breeding attempts. Foal heat (first estrus after birthing) usually occurs between 5 and 13 days post partum. A general rule is to breed every other day based upon standing estrus for three cycles maximum, and if the animal does not conceive or stay pregnant, start looking for the source of the problem. Common reasons for lack of conception may be related to jennet problems such as: uterine infection, stress associated with breeding, or emotional immaturity. It could also be a jack problem with poor semen quality or exhaustion of sperm reserves from overbreeding. The third potential and common problem area is with the people managing the breeding program: handlers should breed the animals at the proper time when the jennet is fully receptive to ensure the best chance of achieving pregnancy. This requires careful and dedicated teasing practices to detect estrus.

Once pregnancy is established, it should continue to be monitored by ultrasound or rectal examination. An ultrasound exam is often performed again at 35–40 days at which time it is easy to identify the fetus and the fetal heartbeat. The rate of twinning in donkeys is reported to be greater than that in horses. Twins should be identified by ultrasound and should be monitored with serial ultrasound exams to follow regression to a singleton if this occurs. If twins persist, then the pregnancy should be terminated with a prostaglandin injection; if allowed to persist, twins are usually aborted in the third trimester or are weak or defective if they survive to term. The donkey placenta is usually not capable of supporting the normal development of two foals.

To ensure that pregnancy is continuing correctly, a third exam may be performed after 90 days. Most early pregnancy loss occurs in the first 90 days. After 90 days, an aborted fetus is often found on the grounds by animal caretakers. The jennet can also be teased periodically to check for sexual receptivity; only in a small percentage of cases will a pregnant female show estrus-like receptivity despite being pregnant.

Some jennets do not show visible evidence of pregnancy until 8–9 months of gestation. Overweight jennets are a particular challenge. Over-conditioning (excess body weight) of the jennet may lead to problems with delivery due to poor muscle tone and poor milk production whereas under-conditioning may cause severe weight loss of the jennet as the foal continues to develop in utero. There is a large increase in fetal size in the last trimester, which puts a significant demand for increased calories on the pregnant jennet. Not being able to meet this demand may result in birth of undersized foals and insufficient milk production for proper growth. Body condition of pregnant animals should be monitored to avoid these problems.

Some jennets show indigestion problems in late pregnancy due to physical pressure on the GI tract. Jennets may also develop extensive edema on the lower body wall—sometimes up to 6 inches thick. Exercise helps to minimize edema so medication is not indicated. Edema usually resolves soon after birth of the foal as the weight of the fetus is removed from the ventral abdomen and circulation is restored in the jennet's tissues.

Pre-Foaling Medical Care

Vaccines should be selected by consulting with the local veterinarian who will recommend products based upon the risk of local diseases, and relative to the safety of specific vaccines indicated for pregnant equines. Those vaccines used in pregnant horses can safely be used in donkeys. These boosters increase circulating antibodies in the dam's system and thereby provide levels in the colostrum (the first milk), which then are available to the foal at the time of first nursing. Immunizations are typically given to the jennet at 4–8 weeks prior to the anticipated birthing and may include Eastern and Western encephalomyelitis, tetanus, influenza, rhinopneumonitis, West Nile virus, and rabies. Deworming of the pregnant jennet should be provided throughout pregnancy depending on the potential for parasite exposure; the products and the frequency given should be decided in consultation with your local veterinarian.

Foaling Process

Normally, the entire foaling process takes approximately 40 minutes from the water breaking to the completion of birth. Once the foal starts to exit the birth canal, there should be progressive exposure of its body with each passing minute. The placentation of the jennet is such that the outer (red) bag ruptures inside the dam and the foal is born inside the inner (translucent white) bag, the *amnion*. If a red bag, the chorioallantoic membrane, is seen protruding from the vulva, then the placenta is separating prematurely or has separated from the lining of the uterus—this compromises blood and oxygen supply of the foal. This is an emergency situation requiring immediate action to rupture the red bag to prevent asphyxiation and death of the foal. If the foaling process is not proceeding as expected, a veterinarian should be called immediately to ensure the best chance of a successful delivery. Jennets foal lying down with the foal emerging front feet first ahead of the nose, in a "diving" position. Once delivered, the hind legs of the foal often remain partially inside the vagina while the jennet rests or until she or the foal attempt to stand. This rest period allows valuable blood to be pumped through the umbilical cord to the foal.

Foaling Sequence

The foaling process proceeds at a fairly rapid rate, with specific progression of events (see figs 9.1–9.15) that are useful for monitoring that all is going as expected.

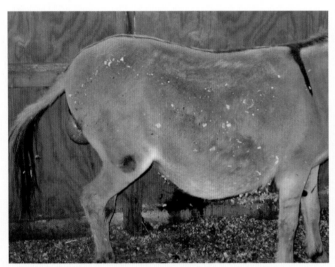

9.1 The inner amniotic sac is protruding from the vulva at the start of delivery.

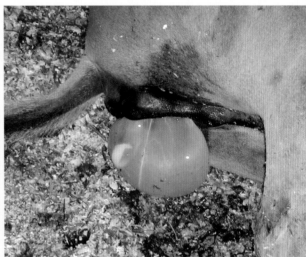

9.2 The jennet is lying down with one foal foot evident.

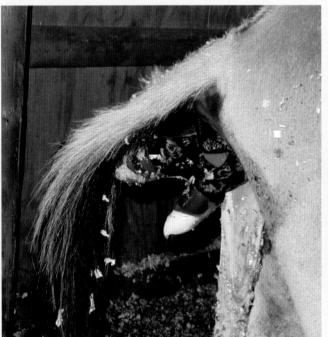

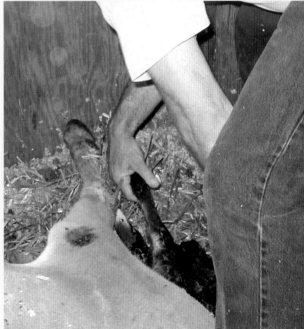

9.5 (Bottom Left) The foaling sac is broken and the jennet is standing up again. You can see the foal's front legs, nose and tongue.

9.6 (Bottom Center) A helper is putting gentle traction on the foal's legs to assist the delivery. Once the foal's shoulders are clear of the vagina, traction should be directed at an angle similar to the position of the jennet's hind legs—that is, down and back.

9.7 (Bottom Right) The front of the foal is out and he is breathing; the jennet is still down.

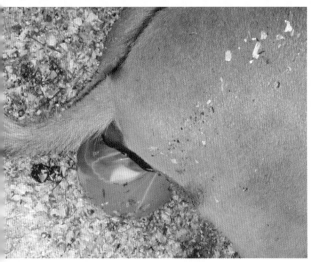

9.3 One foot and the tip of the foal's nose can now be seen.

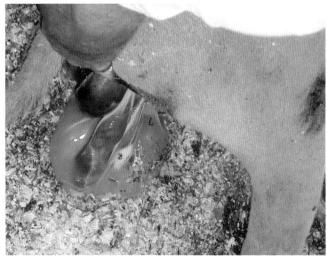

9.4 Both feet and the nose are visible.

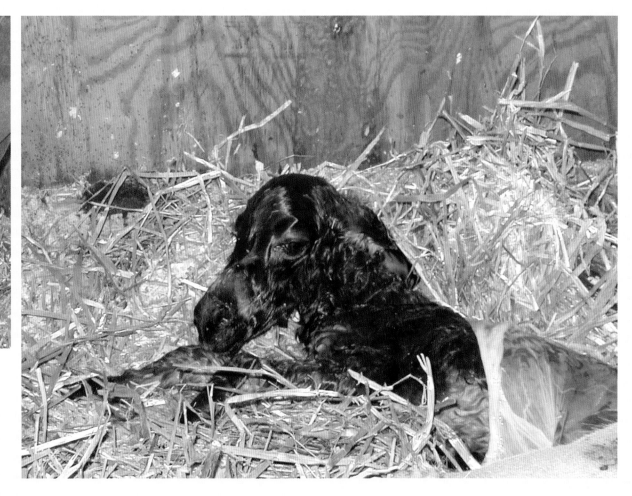

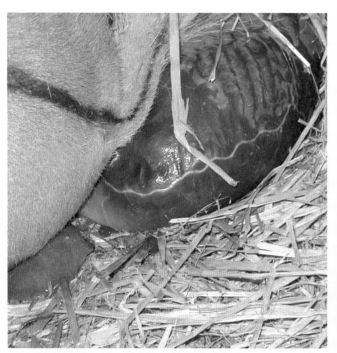

9.8 The hind legs are still inside the jennet while she is down.

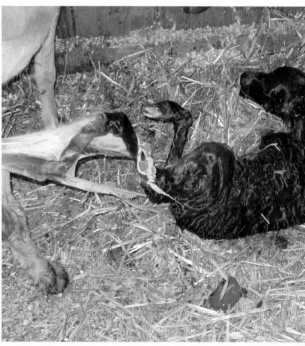

9.9 The jennet stands up allowing the rest of the foal to be delivered and the umbilical cord breaks.

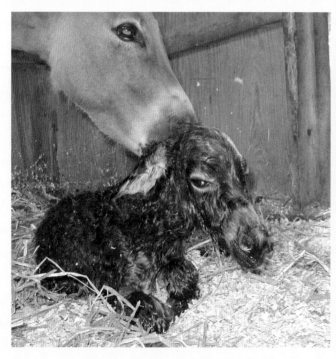

9.12 She licks the foal. He does not appear to be too happy about it!

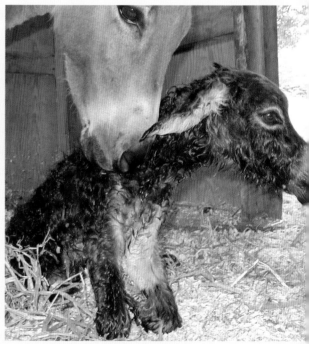

9.13 The foal makes his first attempt to get up.

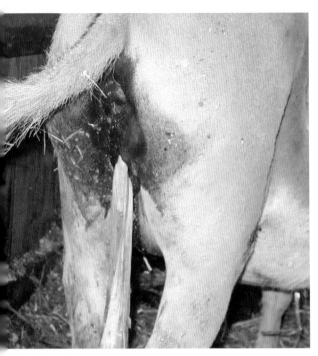

9.10 The placenta is hanging from the jennet's vulva.

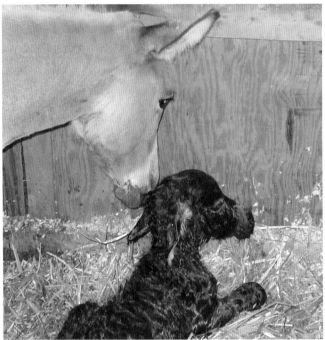

9.11 The jennet smells and bonds with her newborn foal.

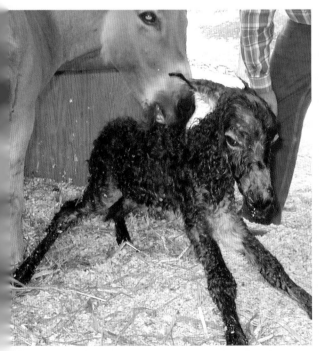

9.14 After a few unsuccessful tries, he gets to his feet.

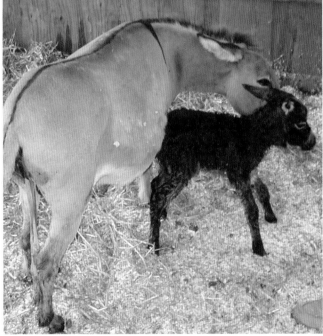

9.15 The jennet and the foal are both standing 15 minutes after he was born.

Immediate Post-Foaling Behavior

The newborn foal breathes immediately after delivery. If any difficulty is noted, then the foal should be held up by the hind legs to allow fluid to drain from the lungs and throat. The nose may also be milked downward and the chest compressed until breathing is steady and the foal is reacting normally.

General rules for newborn foals and jennets:
1. Foal should be standing in 1 hour.
2. Foal should be nursing in 2 hours.
3. Placenta should be passed within 2–3 hours.

If any of the above criteria are not fulfilled, call the vet immediately!

Neonatal Exams of Foals

Normally, the only interventions suggested in newborn foals are to provide protection from adverse weather conditions, to dip the navel in dilute chlorhexidine solution, and to ensure that the jennet and foal bond and the foal successfully nurses. It is best to give the new mother and foal some space and time so as not to interfere with the bonding process. Donkey jennets may foal apart from the herd and keep their foals away from other animals even to the extent of standing out in the rain or snow. Note that winter and early spring weather pose challenges for foaling; during that time, a dry stall should be prepared. It may be necessary to bring the foal inside out of the rain with the jennet following along and to keep them there in sight of other animals initially.

Physical examination of the foal by a veterinarian is usually performed on the day of birth. It includes auscultation of heart, lungs, and abdomen for presence of normal sounds. Normal newborn donkeys may have a systolic heart murmur heard loudest on the left side of the chest due to persistent opening of the lung bypass in the fetal circulation, called *patent ductus arteriosus*. Increasing oxygen in the neonatal blood stream usually results in the closing of this bypass. This murmur should resolve spontaneously by the recheck in three weeks, indicating complete closure of the bypass. If the foal shows evidence of circulatory insufficiency, such as reduced exercise tolerance, lethargy, abnormal mucous membrane color, or delayed capillary refill time, or if the murmur is not gone, a more serious problem should be considered.

The foal's eyes should be clear and he should be stimulated by his surroundings. The umbilicus should be checked for the presence of an opening in the body wall, termed a *hernia*. It is fairly common to feel a defect of one finger diameter at birth but this opening usually closes by 3–4 weeks. If it has not resolved, a veterinarian can use external taping to push the hernial contents into the abdomen—after 2–3 weeks, this defect should then close.

The newborn foal should also be checked for normal limb angulation; many foals may be born with lowered pastern and fetlock angles, which quickly correct spontaneously with time and light exercise. A check of the oral mucosa should reveal normal color and capillary refill time. A jack foal should be checked for the presence of both testicles. If both are not located at birth, then periodic rechecks will verify their presence and proper descent, or not. A jennet foal should be checked for the presence of two teats and a normal vulvar opening. Some practitioners and farm managers routinely administer an enema of 60 cc of warm, soapy water or a Fleet™ enema to all newborn foals in the first day of life to prevent meconium (fecal debris accumulated in the foal during gestation) impaction. Normal nursing of colostrum hydrates the foal and stimulates bowel activity, but an enema does no harm if administered carefully.

Jennet Exam on Foaling Day

Following foaling, the jennet's body condition should be evaluated to determine the need for increasing feed, and her appetite should be robust. Her vulva should be checked for the presence of tears that might need surgical repair; these are uncommon. The udder is checked for the presence of colostrum in both teats. The placenta should pass within 2–3 hours of foaling and it is important to examine it to ensure that it has passed completely. The entire placenta should be spread on the ground to determine if it is fully intact, including all portions of both uterine horns. Any missing piece dictates that this is an emergency situation requiring veterinary medical care to prevent uterine infection (endometritis) and potential laminitis.

It is also important to make sure that the jennet passes manure within the first 24 hours of birthing. A jennet that has had a difficult delivery may have pain in the vulvar and anal areas, making her reluctant to defecate. Pain medication may be indicated in such cases; feeding a bran mash may also improve water intake to soften the manure for easier passage.

Passive Transfer of Maternal Antibodies to the Foal

The foal receives pre-formed antibodies (immunoglobulins) from the jennet by ingesting colostrum. These antibodies are relatively large protein molecules that cross into the circulation from the gut lining for a limited time only, within the initial 24 hours, but usually the majority of this passive transfer of immunoglobulins occurs only during the first 8–12 hours after birth. It is critical that the foal begins to nurse early, within the first couple of hours. These antibodies are the only protection the foal has until his own immune system is able to manufacture antibodies, which does not begin until approximately two months of age.

Evaluation of the success of passive transfer of antibodies in a foal is accomplished by collecting a blood sample after the foal is 8–12 hours old. There are stall-side, field tests that provide rapid results as to the level of immunoglobulin (IgG) a newborn has received. Levels of at least 400 mg/dl of IgG are considered the acceptable minimum for adequate transfer of passive antibodies. If an unacceptable level is determined before the foal is 18–24 hours old, he can be supplemented with thawed, frozen oral colostrum saved from another jennet. If results are not available until after this limited window of opportunity and the IgG level is less than 400 mg/dl, consideration should be given to administering an intravenous plasma transfusion to protect the newborn foal from contracting infectious disease. High-risk foals (premature, sick, or defective) may require a plasma transfusion regardless of the IgG level. This procedure has inherent risk associated with it including infection, anaphylactic shock, and death, and thus its use must be carefully evaluated. If a transfusion is administered the IgG level should be retested 48 hours later to ensure a value greater than 400 mg/dl has been attained.

Lactation and Foal Growth

Normal Donkey Lactation

Normally, the jennet has two functioning teats (nipples). Foals often find the teats without assistance once on their feet. Contractions of the uterus and milk letdown are stimulated by the hormone oxytocin that is released by the jennet as the foal nurses. Antibody-rich colostrum is produced for the first few days, although it cannot be absorbed efficiently by the foal after 12–24 hours. Newborns should be checked to make sure they nurse from both mammary glands; an obvious mismatch in udder size and teat filling is noticeable if this is not happening. A distended udder is susceptible to mastitis (infected or inflamed mammary gland), yet mastitis is uncommon in donkeys.

Insufficient Milk Production

A foal that always seems hungry often indicates that the jennet is not producing sufficient milk. A hungry foal may even approach other mothers to try to nurse. Another sign of poor milk quantity or quality might be a lower than expected growth rate of the foal. Common reasons for milk deficiency include poor nutritional status of the dam, insufficient caloric and protein intake during lactation, or that the dam is a poor milk producer due to genetics—a known poor producer should not be rebred.

Inexperienced mothering behavior of a first time mother may interfere with milk production, as might obesity. Obese jennets have excess fat deposition in the udder, which interferes with mild production. Mastitis, while uncommon, could also decrease milk flow; if present or suspected, systemic antibiotics along with anti-inflammatory medications may be indicated.

Extra milk can be provided with goat milk or equine foal milk replacer to supplement donkey foals whose dams do not produce enough or for orphaned foals. Feedings should be frequent during the first two weeks of life: a general guideline is to feed the foal an amount equivalent to 10–12% of its body weight, splitting the meals into six feedings throughout the day. A pint of milk weighs 1 lb, so a 60 lb donkey foal receives approximately 6 pints per day in divided feedings. It is not necessary to wake a foal during the middle of the night for feeding—that is sleep time. Supplemental feeding frequency may be decreased steadily to twice daily by the first eight weeks of life.

A dam that has been on an insufficient diet during and/or following pregnancy can be helped by providing her with free-choice, quality grass hay, clean, fresh water (warmed in winter to encourage consumption), and supplementation with free-choice, balanced minerals. A supplemental source of calories and protein such as 1:1 parts cracked corn to soybean meal may be provided to dams in poor body condition. Equine pelleted feeds formulated for lactating mares can also be used. The donkey foal begins eating solid food within a week or two, sharing with the mother. The foal may be offered similar nutritional choices as the dam by using a creep feeder that allows the foal access to the food at will without having to compete with larger animals or other adults.

Lack of Foal Weight Gain

There are no published studies that define normal growth rates for donkey foals. This characteristic is closely tied to genetics and also the available food supply for dam and foal. A foal can be compared to others of the same age and size or weight. This provides a check for inadequate growth that may be related to deficiencies in the dam, such as poor milk production or limited mammary gland capacity, or insufficient access to good quality food. Some foals flourish well up to about 2 months and then growth stalls as the dam's milk production no longer supports normal, continued growth of the foal.

Growth deficiency in the foal may be caused by an infection (bacterial or parasitic), not enough calories, or limited access to food. A fecal examination is used to check for internal parasites; appropriate parasite control measures can then be taken (see p. 38). Some foals are just poor doers from the start. It is important to correct nutritional deficiencies in slow-growing foals, including problems with accessibility to feed. It might be best to put the foal and dam into a small feeding group or separate them so they do not have to contend with herd competition for food or water.

Guidelines for Foals and Rebreeding Jennets

A jennet may exhibit *lactational anestrus* (absence of the heat cycle) and not show signs of heat while nursing a foal. She may also be protective of her foal when teased or approached by a jack and it may be necessary to move the foal a short distance away (but still in her visual field) for her to show interest in the jack. It is a good idea to allow foals to see the breeding process so that it is not foreign to them should they be used for breeding later.

A foal born to a jennet that was well-immunized prior to foaling may be started on a vaccination program for encephalitis, West Nile virus, rabies, and tetanus at 3–5 months of age with a booster administered one month later. The respiratory vaccine series is begun at approximately the same age. If the foal was born to a non-vaccinated jennet, all immunizations should begin at 3–4 months of age. Many owners deworm foals monthly through

6 months of age, starting at 8 weeks of age. Care must be taken not to over-dose young foals as some medications have narrow margins of safety (see chapter 4, p. 30).

Weaning the Foal

There are many opinions as to *how*, *when*, or even *if* weaning should be done. Donkeys are herd animals with a well-defined social structure. A slow weaning process is recommended for foals rather than an abrupt separation—this reduces stress and the risk of injury to a distressed foal or jennet that try to reunite.

At 4–6 months of age, the foal may be stalled next to its mother at night and then gradually kept separated for longer periods over the next several weeks until the weaning process is completed. Some owners elect not to wean female foals, preferring to leave them with their mothers who eventually self-wean them.

9.16 An Asian Wild Ass (Kulan) jennet and her foal.

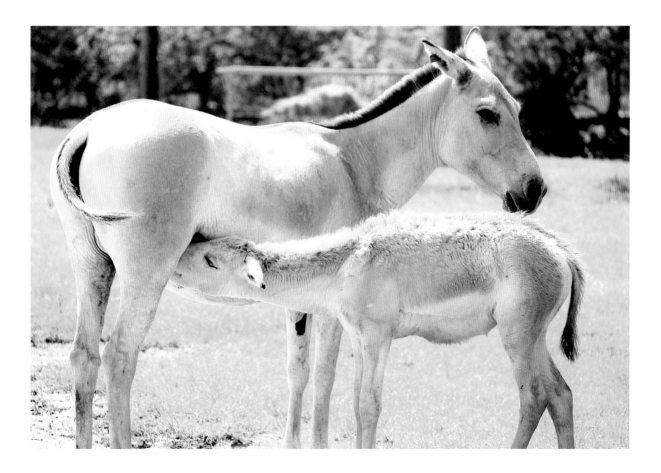

A jack foal is usually weaned from his dam by 6 months of age, using the gradual weaning process. Young jacks should be removed from the vicinity of female donkeys as they are capable of impregnating jennets by 8 months of age. A precocious jack foal may be injured if he tries to mount an aggressive jennet. Play mounting behavior is seen in some very young jacks, most often directed toward their mothers. The jennet will correct an aggressive foal by biting or kicking in reprimand.

Summary

- Gestational length in the donkey is approximately 12–13 months with some researchers reporting an average length of 372–374 days. Pregnancy confirmation using standard ultrasound equipment can begin at 16 days following breeding with additional ultrasounds beginning at 25–28 days of gestation. By this time, based on an average estrus cycle of 28 days, the jennet should either be pregnant or have returned to estrus.

- A general rule is to breed three times and if the animal does not conceive or stay pregnant, start looking for the source of the problem. Common reasons for lack of conception may be related to jennet problems, jack problems, or problems with the people managing the breeding program.

- Over-conditioning (excess body weight) of the jennet may lead to problems with delivery due to poor muscle tone and poor milk production, whereas under-conditioning may cause severe weight loss of the jennet as the foal continues to develop in utero.

- There is a large increase in fetal size in the last trimester of pregnancy, which puts a significant demand for increased calories on the pregnant jennet. Not being able to meet this demand may result in birth of an undersized foal and insufficient milk production for proper growth. Body condition of pregnant animals should be monitored to avoid these problems.

- Pre-foaling medical care for jennets includes use of appropriate immunizations and deworming medications as indicated by fecal examination.

- The foaling process proceeds at a fairly rapid rate, with specific progression of events that are useful for monitoring that all is going as expected.

- Jennets foal lying down with the foal emerging front feet first ahead of the nose, in a "diving" position. Once delivered, the hind legs of the foal often remain partially inside the vagina while the jennet rests or until she or the foal attempt to stand.

- The newborn foal breathes immediately after delivery. If any difficulty is noted, then the foal should be held up by the hind legs to allow fluid to drain from the lungs and throat. The nose may also be "milked" downward and the chest compressed until breathing is steady and the foal is reacting normally.

- General rules for newborn foals and jennets: standing in 1 hour, nursing in 2 hours, and placenta passed within 2–3 hours.

- Normally, the only interventions suggested in newborn foals are to provide protection from adverse weather conditions; to dip the navel in dilute chlorhexidine solution; and to ensure that the jennet and foal bond and the foal successfully nurses. It is best to give the new mother and foal some space and time so as not to interfere with the bonding process.

- The foal receives preformed antibodies (immunoglobulins) from the jennet by ingesting colostrum. These antibodies are relatively large protein molecules that cross into the circulation from the gut lining for a limited time only—within the initial 24 hours, but usually the majority of this passive transfer of immunoglobulins occurs only during the first 8–12 hours after birth.

- It is critical that the foal begins to nurse early, within the first couple of hours. These antibodies are the only protection the foal has until its immune system is able to manufacture its own antibodies, which does not begin until approximately 2 months of age.

- High-risk foals (premature, sick, or defective) may require a plasma transfusion regardless of the IgG level to provide sufficient protective antibodies.

- Newborns should be checked to make sure they nurse from both mammary glands; an obvious mismatch in udder size and teat filling is noticeable if this is not happening. A distended udder is susceptible to mastitis (infected or inflamed mammary gland), yet mastitis is uncommon in donkeys.

- A foal that always seems hungry often indicates that the jennet is not producing sufficient milk. A hungry foal may even approach other mothers to try to nurse. Another sign of poor milk quantity or quality might be a lower than expected growth rate of the foal.

- Common reasons for milk deficiency include poor nutritional status of the dam; insufficient caloric and protein intake during lactation; or that the dam is a poor milk producer due to genetics—a known poor producer should not be rebred.

- A jennet may exhibit lactational anestrus and not show signs of heat while nursing a foal. She may also be protective of her foal when teased or approached by a jack and it may be necessary to move the foal a short distance away (but still in her visual field) for her to show interest in the jack. It is a good idea to allow foals to see the breeding process so that it is not foreign to them should they used for breeding later.

- There are many opinions as to *how*, *when*, or even *if* weaning of foals should be done. A slow weaning process is recommended for foals rather than an abrupt separation—this reduces stress and the risk of injury to a distressed foal or jennet that try to reunite.

References

1. Pugh, DG. "Donkey Reproduction." Proceedings of the Annual Convention of the AAEP. 2002; 113-114.

Appendix A
Normal Physical Exam Parameters

Body Temperature

Adult Donkey   36.2–37.8 (average 37.1) °C
                  97.2–100.0 (average 98.8) °F

Young Donkey   36.6–38.9 (average 37.6) °C
                  97.8–102.1 (average 99.6) °F

Pulse Rate

Adult Donkey   36–68 (average 44) beats per minute
Young Donkey   44–80 (average 60) beats per minute

Respiratory Rate

Adult Donkey   12–44 (average 20) breaths per minute
Young Donkey   16–48 (average 28) breaths per minute

Reference

Svendsen, E. *The Professional Handbook of the Donkey*. 3rd edition. The Donkey
  Sanctuary, 1997.

Appendix B

Reference Ranges for Blood Hemogram and Serum Chemistry Tests

Donkey Hemogram Test	Units	Normal Range	Comments
Red Blood Cells (RBC)	$X10^6/\mu L$	4.6–9.0	2
Hemoglobin (Hb)	g/dl	9.5–16.5	2
Packed Cell Volume (PCV)	%	28.0–48.0	2
Mean Corpuscular Volume (MCV)	fl	46.5–68.0	2
Mean Corpuscular Hemoglobin Concentration (MCHC)	g/dl	32.0–36.5	2
Mean Corpuscular Hemoglobin (MCH)	pg	16.0–23.5	2
Platelets	$X10^3/\mu l$	160–580	3
White Blood Cells (WBC)	$X10^3/\mu l$	5.2–15.5	4
Band Neutrophils (Bands)	%	0.0–1.0	4
	$X10^3/\mu l$	0.0–100.0	
Neutrophils	%	23.0–76.0	4
	$X10^3/\mu l$	1.5–10.0	
Lymphocytes	%	14.5–65.0	4
	$X10^3/\mu l$	1.1–7.5	
Monocytes	%	0.0–11.5	4
	$X10^3/\mu l$	0–1100	
Eosinophils	%	0.0–15.0	4
	$X10^3/\mu l$	0–1650	
Basophils	%	0.0–1.5	4
	$X10^3/\mu l$	0–175	4
Neutrophils:Lymphocytes		0.0–1.5	4
Icterus Index		2–5	5
Plasma Protein	g/dl	6.0–8.5	6
Fibrinogen	mg/dl	100–500	7

Donkey Serum Chemistry Test	Units	Normal Range	Comments
Serum Protein	g/dl	5.5–8.5	6
Albumin	g/dl	2.5–4.0	8
Globulin	g/dl	2.5–5.5	9
Albumin:Globulin Ratio		0.5–1.5	16
Total Bilirubin	mg/dl	0.0–0.5	10
Blood Urea Nitrogen (BUN)	mg/dl	7–25	11
Creatinine	mg/dl	0.6–1.6	12

Glucose	mg/dl	40–130	13
Cholesterol	mg/dl	50–170	10
Creatine Phosphokinase (CK or CPK)	U/L	20–170	14
Aspartate Aminotransferase (AST)	U/L	250–725	17
Alanine Aminotransferase (ALT)	U/L	0–70	18
Sorbitol Dehydrogenease (SDH)	U/L	0.2–6.0	19
Alkaline Phosphatase (ALP or AP)	U/L	90–400	20
Gamma Glutamyl Transferase (GGT)	U/L	10–130	21
Lactate Dehydrogenase (LDH)	U/L	105–750	10, 14
Inorganic Phosphorus	mg/dl	1.8–7.0	12, 22
Calcium	mg/dl	10.0–13.0	23
Magnesium	mg/dl	1.8–3.6	
Sodium	mEq/L	132–148	24
Potassium	mEq/L	2.5–5.4	25
Chloride	mEq/L	95–109	26

Comments

1. Values are adapted from Zinkl, JG, et al, "Reference Ranges and the Influence of Age and Sex on Hematological and Serum Biochemical Values in Donkeys (*Equus asinus*)," *American Journal of Veterinary Research*, 51:3, 408-413, 1990. They were derived from 217 donkeys, both feral and domestic, sampled in California.

2. Used to evaluate anemia and the body's response to it.

3. Used to evaluate ability of blood to clot.

4. Used to evaluate shifts in numbers and types of white blood cells seen in various diseases.

5. Indicator of red blood cell breakdown and liver function.

6. Used to evaluate dehydration, nutritional status, and response to disease.

7. Increased in chronic inflammatory disease.

8. The major serum protein—decreased in liver disease and malnutrition.

9. Increased in chronic immune system stimulation, e.g., infections.

10. May be increased with liver disease.

11. May be decreased with liver disease and increased with kidney disease.

12. May be increased with kidney disease.

13. May be increased with stress or Cushing's disease and diabetes, and decreased with malnutrition.

14. May be increased with muscle disease or damage.

15. Levels are influenced by bone damage and turnover.

16. Decreased with excess globulin production as a result of antigenic stimulation.

17. Increased usually as a result of liver or muscle injury.

18. Increased usually as a result of muscle injury.

19. Increased with liver damage only.

20. Found in liver, bone, and placenta.

21. Associated with liver cells and biliary cells.

22. Decreased with inadequate intake or intestinal malabsorption.

23. Increased with neoplasia, renal failure, bone lysis, and Vitamin D toxicosis. Decreased in malabsorption, dietary insufficiency, or sweating.

24. Essential for renal water retention to control hydration status. May be decreased with diarrhea, saliva loss, sweating, or inadequate intake. May be increased with lack of water or by high salt diet with restricted water intake.

25. Necessary for proper cardiac and neuromuscular function. May be increased with marked muscle exertion, renal disease, and urinary obstruction. May be decreased with anorexia, diarrhea, profuse sweating, and prolonged exercise.

26. An important component of gastric fluid, sweat, and saliva. Usually varies in parallel with sodium.

Additional Comments:

Age influences:

a. Eosinophil counts, MCV, MCH, and plasma protein, serum protein, and serum globulin concentrations increase with age.

b. Erythrocyte (RBC) and platelet counts and fibrinogen, glucose, and potassium concentrations decrease with age.

c. Lymphocyte counts decrease with age probably reflecting the progressive development of the immune system in younger animals.

d. Alkaline phosphatase decreases with age.

e. Eosinophil counts increase with age perhaps as a result of increasing intestinal parasite burdens.

f. Inorganic phosphorus decreases with age probably reflecting decreased bone metabolism.

Sex influences:

a. MCH is higher in females.

b. Female donkeys have significantly higher MCHC and leukocyte (WBC) and neutrophil counts than male donkeys.

Feral donkeys have lower levels of eosinophilic blood cells possibly indicating less intestinal parasite infection, or it may be associated with the stress of capture.

Serum LDH is higher in miniature donkeys than in other donkeys.

Working donkeys may have lower sodium levels than resting donkeys due to loss from sweating.

Differences from horses:

a. Donkeys have fewer but larger RBCs.

b. Icterus index and bilirubin concentration are lower in donkeys.

c. Serum CPK and GGT are higher in donkeys.

Additional Reference

Latimer, KS, Mahaffey, EA, and Prasse KW. *Veterinary Laboratory Medicine: Clinical Pathology.* Iowa State University Press, 2003.

Donkey Organizations

American Donkey and Mule Society
P.O. Box 1210
Lewisville, TX 75067
www.lovelongears.com

National Miniature Donkey Association
1450 Dewey Road
Rome, NY 13440
www.nmdaasset.com

Canadian Donkey and Mule Association
Box 341
Nanton, Alberta, Canada
T0L1R0
www.donkeyandmule.com

American Council of Spotted Asses
Box 121
New Meile, MO 63365
www.spottedass.com

Animal Traction Network for Eastern and
Southern Africa (ATNESA)
www.atnesa.org
(The ATNESA seeks to improve information exchange
regarding animal draft power and documents re-
sources by country and region for the entire world.)

Donkey Publications

The Brayer Magazine
(see American Donkey and Mule Society)

Asset
(see National Miniature Donkey Association)

Mules and More Magazine
P.O. Box 460
Bland, MO 65014
www.mulesandmore.com

Textbooks

Hutchins, Betsy and Paul. *The Definitive Donkey:
A Textbook on the Modern Ass.* Hee Haw Book
Service, 1999.

Svendsen, Elisabeth D. *The Professional Handbook of the Donkey.* Whittet Books,1997.

Glossary

Abdominocentesis The process of obtaining a sample of the abdominal fluid for analysis.

Alveoli Small air sacs in the lungs.

Analgesic Pain relieving medication.

Anorexia Lack of appetite, also known as inappetance.

Anthelmentics Drugs that are used to treat parasitic worms.

Articular Referring to the joint.

Articular cartilage Joint cartilage located on the ends of bones that contact each other—it helps bone movement.

Ataxia Incoordination.

Auscultation The act of listening to sounds arising within organs (the lungs or heart, for example) as an aid to diagnosis and treatment.

Avermectin compound Anthelmintic drugs with the chemical structure of avermectins.

Biopsy Piece of tissue submitted for microscopic examination of its structure.

Bot Stomach larva of flies of the bot family.

Buccal cavity Mouth cavity.

Capsulitis Inflammation of the joint capsule.

Cellulitis Inflammation of the tissues.

Cellulose A polysaccharide (complex sugar) $(C_6H_{10}O_5)x$ made up of glucose; it constitutes the chief part of the cell walls of plants.

Coprophagy Eating of feces.

Crepitus A grating or crackling sound or sensation (as that produced by the fractured ends of a bone moving against each other or joints with severe arthritic boney changes).

Cushing's disease A disease of the pituitary gland in equines resulting in excessive cortisol production by the adrenal glands; long hair coat inappropriate to environmental temperatures; increased sweating; muscle wasting; increased urination and water consumption; and possibly resulting in immunosuppression and laminitis.

Cytology The study of cells.

Deciduous teeth Nonpermanent teeth that are normally shed as the permanent teeth erupt.

Dental points Sharp edges that develop on the outsides of the upper cheek teeth and insides of the lower cheek teeth as a result of chewing only soft feeds; these points may need to be removed by "floating" of the teeth with a dental file.

Digital Referring to the foot.

Dystocia Abnormal birth; birthing difficulty.

Eclampsia Weakness, coma, or convulsions associated with low blood calcium.

Endemic Restricted or peculiar to a locality or region.

Endometritis Inflammation of the lining of the uterus (endometrium).

Endotoxemia A poisonous substance (toxin) in the blood, which is released from the bacterial cell body upon its disintegration.

Eosinophils White blood cells with cytoplasmic inclusions readily stained red by eosin.

Epidemic A disease that affects an atypically large number of individuals within a population, community, or region, suddenly and at the same time.

Epiphysis A part of a bone that ossifies separately and later becomes fused to the main part of the bone, as at the end of a long bone.

Equids Members of the family Equidae, such as donkeys, horses, and mules.

Estrus A regularly recurrent state of sexual excitability during which the female equine will accept the male and is capable of conceiving.

Etiology The cause or causes of a disease or abnormal condition.

Fecalith A concretion of dry compact feces formed in the intestine.

Founder To become disabled or to go lame, especially in association with laminitis.

Gestation Pregnancy.

Heart murmur Abnormal heart sound caused by turbulent blood flow.

Hemicellulose Any of various plant polysaccharides less complex than cellulose and easily hydrolyzable to simple sugars and other products.

Hernia A protrusion of an organ or part through connective tissue or through the wall of the cavity in which it is normally enclosed.

Hyperlipemia Increased fat in the blood.

Hypersecretion Increased secretion such as occurs in some forms of diarrhea within the intestinal tract.

Hypobiosis A low energy or inactive state of a living organism such as in the case of small strongyles within the walls of the intestinal tract.

Ileus A failure of peristalsis within the gastrointestinal (GI) tract resulting in backup of intestinal contents.

Inappetance Lack of appetite, also known as anorexia.

Inflammation Abnormal tissue appearance and function characterized by heat, pain, swelling, redness, and loss of function.

Lactational anestrus Lack of estrus cycling due to nursing a foal.

Laminae The sensitive tissues within the hoof that connect and suspend the pedal bone to the inside of the hoof wall.

Laminitis Inflammation of the lamina in the hoof, typically caused by excessive ingestion of a dietary substance (as carbohydrate)—also known as founder.

Lubricin A lubricating protein physiologically present in the synovial fluid, which reduces friction and prevents wear and tear at the cartilage surface.

Lymphatic A vessel that contains or conveys lymph; it originates as an interfibrillar or intercellular cleft or space in a tissue or organ. If small it has no distinct walls or walls composed only of endothelial cells, and if large it resembles a vein in structure.

Malabsorption Improper absorption of digested substances from the gastrointestinal (GI) tract.

Maldigestion Improper digestion of food stuffs in the GI tract.

Mandible The upper jaw bone.

Maxilla The lower jaw bone.

Meconium The newborn foal's first stool, which can result in a painful impaction if it is not passed.

Medial saphenous vein The large superficial vein on the inside of the hind leg.

Microflora The microorganisms (bacteria or fungi) living in or on the body in a localized region, such as the intestinal microflora.

Monogastric Animal having a single-compartment stomach.

Monosaccharide A simple sugar not decomposable to simpler sugars by hydrolysis.

Morbidity Sickness.

Mortality Death.

Mucosa A membrane rich in mucous glands; specifically one that lines body passages and cavities that communicate directly or indirectly with the exterior (such as the alimentary, respiratory, and genitourinary tracts). It functions in protection, support, nutrient absorption, and secretion of mucus, enzymes, and salts.

Mycotoxins Toxins produced by fungi.

Occlusal surfaces of the teeth The surfaces that oppose and contact each other during mastication (chewing).

Oribatid forage mite A small mite found on pasture, which serves as the intermediate host of the donkey tapeworm.

Osteoarthritis Arthritis typically with onset during middle or old age that is characterized by degenerative and sometimes hypertrophic changes in the bone and cartilage of one or more joints and a progressive wearing down of apposing joint surfaces with consequent distortion of joint position; it is characterized by pain, swelling, and stiffness.

Osteochondrosis A bone and cartilage maturation defect that may result in arthritis and lameness.

Palmar Referring to the back of the foreleg.

Patent infection Infection characterized by shedding of infectious particles.

Pathogenic Disease causing.

PDA Patent ductus arteriosus. In the developing fetus, the ductus arteriosus (DA) is a shunt connecting the pulmonary artery to the aortic arch that allows most of the blood from the right ventricle to bypass the fetus' fluid-filled lungs.

Percussion Production of a sound by any action that sets the object into vibration, such as tapping the abdomen with a finger while simultaneously listening to the adjacent area with a stethoscope; used to detect abnormal sound transmission in a portion of the body from the outside.

Peristalsis Successive waves of involuntary contraction, which pass along the walls of a hollow muscular structure (such as the esophagus or intestine) and force the contents onward.

Physis The region in a long bone between the epiphysis and diaphysis where growth in length occurs; the growth plate.

Physitis/epiphysitis Inflammation of the growth plate/epiphysis of a bone.

Plantar Referring to the back of the hind leg.

Quidding/cudding Dropping food from the mouth while chewing.

Rhabdomyolysis A destructive muscle condition associated with heat exhaustion. It can lead to renal failure, indicated by dark-colored urine from muscle cell breakdown pigments, and fluid congestion of the heart and lungs.

Sodium hyaluronate (hyaluronic acid) A major component of the synovial fluid; found to increase the viscosity of the fluid. Along with lubricin, it is one of the fluid's main lubricating components. It is an important component of articular cartilage, where it is present as a coat around each cell (chondrocyte) improving its resistance to compression.

Strongyle A nematode worm of the family *Strongylidae*, order *Strongylida*. They are often parasitic in the gastrointestinal tract of mammals, especially equines.

Subchondral bone Bone located just below the articular cartilage, which provides its support.

Synovial fluid The viscous lubricating fluid secreted by the cells (synovial cells or synoviocytes), which line the inside of a synovial joint.

Synovitis Inflammation of the synovial tissue inside the joint.

Toxemia The presence of toxins in the blood.

Transabdominal ultrasound exam Examination of the internal structures of the abdomen using an ultrasound probe applied to the abdominal wall.

Transrectal ultrasound exam Examination of the internal abdominal structures using an ultrasound probe inserted into the rectum as in examination of the female internal genital organs or the urinary bladder.

Viremia Virus in the blood.

Index